"What this book accurately calls the 'horror' of the HIV epidemic is fading from memory. The authors have salvaged what needs to be remembered and learned from the experience of those for whom the horror was every day, lived reality."

Jonathan Grimshaw, MBE, Activist

"Seen through the eyes of people who lived it, this unique account of four decades of HIV in the UK is part oral history and part analysis of responses to the personal, medical, and social challenges the epidemic imposed. It offers much wisdom and useful lessons for the future of humane and person-centred models of care, in pandemics and beyond."

Hilary Curtis, PhD, Freelance Researcher

"Eloquent and a mix of painful and inspiring, this book, assembled from a group of seemingly disparate but deeply interconnected actors, tells stories of suffering, mobilisation and hope. It is a form of remembrance, but it is also much more. It is an account of trauma and atrocity, understanding and advocacy, as well as partnership and collaboration. Now, more than ever, we need these rigorous, critical studies that foster a collective memory around how epidemics are iteratively experienced, managed, and overcome."

Professor Alex Broom, Professor of Sociology, School of Social and Political Sciences, University of Sydney, NSW

"Passionate, poignant, inspiring and timely. This excellent book recounts the experiences of those on the front line of the epidemic over the past four decades. This is history. A tribute to those who have died … and to those living with HIV today."

Christopher Sandford, Theatre and Film Director and Activist

"This is a compelling story of HIV and AIDS that does justice to the emotions, the fears, and the hopes of the patients and health care workers who together fought battles for social justice, medical advances, compassion, and holistic care. The partnership between patients and their carers, staff in the NHS and voluntary sectors as well as politicians and the media, was at times fraught and raw, but our learning and reflection of those times can help shape our approaches and aid recovery from current and future challenges of infectious diseases."

Professor Simon Barton, Medical Director of Commissioning, NHSE/I London Region, and HIV/GUM Physician (1988-2020), Chelsea and Westminster Hospital, London

"None of us who lived through the early years of the AIDS crisis could have realised quite how bad things would get, or how long it would last. The authors of this timely book have marshalled a wealth of voices, including doctors, nurses and other carers, activists, and patients, providing vivid personal testimony to the history of HIV/AIDS in the UK, which has until now been significantly neglected.

There are many lessons to be learned from these pages, not the least of which is the role of the state in adequately funding and maintaining public health."

Simon Watney, PLWH, Art Historian and Author

"This is an excellent and much needed book - it is certainly heartfelt, and the quotes are very much the meat of the text. It should be available in schools, colleges, public libraries, and for those on the gay scene and also for medical students and the wider profession, since the lessons learnt here spill over into general medical practice."

Mr Jeremy Booth, Former Clinical Director of Surgery and Accident and Emergency Medicine, Chelsea and Westminster Hospital, London

"The authors have done an extraordinary exploration into the experience of people who lived with the initial shock of AIDS and the subsequent traumas in a health care system and society quite unprepared for the revolution it would create in all sectors. This book is an important insight into the perils of the time and the changes that resulted. Crises drive political change and energise creativity. This book should be a reminder not only that a great deal of suffering brought about these changes but that HIV prevention is still required."

Professor Roy Robertson, GP in Edinburgh and Researcher at Edinburgh University

HIV in the UK

This book explores the thoroughly human dimension of the health care and prevention responses to the HIV crisis in the UK, and the impact that such initiatives had on the progression of the epidemic.

This book presents a compelling account of the unfolding of the epidemic and the initiatives that made all the difference in the care and prevention of HIV in the UK from the early 1980s to the present time. Drawing on interviews with people with HIV, doctors and nurses involved in their care, leaders of AIDS charities, activists, and politicians, it identifies and describes the models of care developed in response to the onset of the HIV epidemic, and its impact on NHS and voluntary organisations. It goes on to explore the political responses, the evolution of HIV stigma, and the personal impact of the early high mortality rates. Finally, it discusses recent organisational changes in the provision of care and prevention services. In doing so, this volume identifies the lessons learnt from the care and prevention of HIV, both in relation to HIV infection and other conditions, such as COVID-19, and discusses future challenges.

This book will be of great value to those working in services dealing with HIV, charities, and Clinical Commissioning Groups and GP organisations, as well as social historians and medical sociologists.

Dr Jose Catalan is a psychiatrist and academic who has held academic posts at the University of Oxford and Imperial College London, and as consultant psychiatrist at Central North West London NHS Foundation Trust. His area of interest is the relationship between physical disorders and mental health problems.

Dr Barbara Hedge is a consultant clinical and health psychologist who specialises in difficulties related to HIV and sexual health. She was Director of the Clinical Psychology training programme at the University of Hertfordshire UK, and Professor of Clinical Psychology at the University of Waikato, NZ.

Professor Damien Ridge is Research Director at the College of Liberal Arts & Sciences, University of Westminster, specialising in chronic health conditions, and is a practising psychotherapist. He has held research posts at the University of Oxford and City University, London.

Routledge Studies in the Sociology of Health and Illness

For more information about this series, please visit: https://www.routledge.com/Routledge-Studies-in-the-Sociology-of-Health-and-Illness/book-series/RSSHI

HIV in the UK

Voices from the Epidemic

**Jose Catalan, Barbara Hedge and
Damien Ridge**

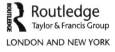 Routledge
Taylor & Francis Group

LONDON AND NEW YORK

First published 2021
by Routledge
2 Park Square, Milton Park, Abingdon, Oxon OX14 4RN

and by Routledge
52 Vanderbilt Avenue, New York, NY 10017

Routledge is an imprint of the Taylor & Francis Group, an informa business

British Library Cataloguing-in-Publication Data
A catalogue record for this book is available from the British Library

Library of Congress Cataloging-in-Publication Data
Names: Catalán, José, 1949- author. | Hedge, Barbara, author. | Ridge, Damien, author.
Title: HIV in the UK : voices from the eipidemic Jose Catalan, Barbara Hedge, and Damien Ridge.
Description: Abingdon, Oxon ; New York, NY : Routledge, 2021. | Series: Routledge studies in the sociology of health and illness | Includes bibliographical references and index.
Identifiers: LCCN 2020034911 (print) | LCCN 2020034912 (ebook) | ISBN 9781138394551 (hardback) | ISBN 9780367682460 (paperback) | ISBN 9780429401107 (ebook)
Subjects: LCSH: AIDS (Disease)--Great Britain. | HIV infections--Great Britian--Prevention. | Strategic planning--Great Britain.
Classification: LCC RA644.A25 C3724 2021 (print) | LCC RA644.A25 (ebook) | DDC 362.19697/9200941--dc23
LC record available at https://lccn.loc.gov/2020034911
LC ebook record available at https://lccn.loc.gov/2020034912

ISBN: 978-1-138-39455-1 (hbk)
ISBN: 978-0-367-68246-0 (pbk)
ISBN: 978-0-429-40110-7 (ebk)

Typeset in Bembo
by SPi Global, India

Contents

Foreword

The COVID-19 pandemic of 2020 has regularly been called the worst global health threat since the Spanish flu epidemic of 1918–19. Somehow the collective historic memory has glossed over a more recent global threat, the HIV/AIDS pandemic from the early 1980s, which despite tremendous medical advances still affects millions of people worldwide. Globally there have been over 75 million cases, and 32 million people have died.

HIV in the UK: Voices from the Epidemic reminds us how easy it is to forget, and how important it is to remember. It is a timely and moving anatomy of the devastation caused by HIV in the UK, but also a tribute to the response it has evoked. It was the first epidemic in which those most affected by it took the lead in combatting it, and in doing so helped transform social, cultural, sexual, and health practices, and created a powerful and lasting legacy. We have done this despite the prejudice, discrimination, fear, ideological and theological denunciations, and moral panic that people living with HIV, and people who died with it, have had to endure.

The problem from the first warnings of an impending crisis in the USA in the summer of 1981 was that a disease (that was not then known as HIV or AIDS) was seen as the disease of marginalised people, and especially gay men. In a climate of heightened political, cultural and moral conflict, and growing reaction to the advances made by LGBT+ people, those most affected by HIV were in effect blamed for it: 'they brought it on themselves'. COVID-19 however was immediately seen as a universal threat: everyone was at risk. Whole societies went into lock-down. Only as the epidemic spread was it belatedly recognised that in fact it differentially affected varying groups of people. In the case of HIV, it was the other way around. Originally classed as the 'gay plague', and then a threat only to the three H's – Homosexuals, Haitians, and Haemophiliacs – it was only when it became seen as a universal threat to the population, that is, the heterosexual population, that governments began to respond in a serious way. And in becoming a universal threat, there was soon a real possibility that the particular needs of marginalised groups would be ignored again. The epidemic in the global north had to be 're-gayed', whilst the needs of other deeply affected, often racialised and minoritised groups had to be constantly reasserted.

But it was those same people living with, and dying from, HIV who forged a way through this historic scandal and tragedy: through innovative forms of mobilisation, collective endeavour, community building, prevention strategies, alliances with public health officials, medics, and scientists, experiments with new modes of medical and community care, treatment activism, new ways of delivering palliative care and thinking about death, transnational alliances, building grass roots knowledge, re-shaping identities, and changing the languages which had demeaned those devastated by the virus into a language of affirmation and hope.

AIDS activists proclaimed that Silence = Death. This book reminds us that Talking = Life. And by giving voice to those who lived through the HIV/AIDS epidemic, as survivors, activists, campaigners, volunteers, professionals, researchers, and the like, all of which are in any case overlapping categories, *HIV in the UK: Voices from the Epidemic* reminds us again that the worst thing we can do is to forget. Those who forget the past may have the misfortune to relive it.

When the HIV/AIDS epidemic burst onto the world stage in the early 1980s, people spoke of how this shouldn't have happened in the modern world. Scientific advances, health improvements, drug therapies had surely ended for ever the pre-modern scourge of the epidemic. This was not true even then. But forty years on, as epidemics of various sorts have swept many parts of the world, they must surely have put paid to such airy optimism. HIV, like COVID-19, reminded us of our vulnerabilities, of the precariousness of everyday life when confronted by the unknown unknowns of a threatened nature. Yet each time we humans are threatened by a new challenge from microscopic bugs we seem to need to re-learn the lessons. It is easy to forget. The voices recorded in this book help us to recognise again how important memory is. Memory is not about something that happened in the past. It is about how we live the present, and face the unknowable future. Which is why it is so important to hear again the voices from the HIV/AIDS epidemic.

Jeffrey Weeks
Emeritus Professor of Sociology, London South Bank University

Acknowledgements

We were inspired and encouraged by the dedication and hard work of people with HIV, activists, and healthcare workers we have known over the years, many of whom sadly have not survived to benefit from the advances made in HIV care and prevention. They all provided us with the determination to ensure that their experiences, actions, and commitment will never be forgotten.

The voices of the participants who were interviewed for the project form the backbone of the book. Together with a number of participants who, for personal reasons, provided anonymous accounts, we are very grateful to everyone who agreed to be interviewed, including:

Michael Adler, Tristan Barber, Simon Barton, Ravneet Batra, Martha Baillie, Ray Brettle, Sharron Brown, Jane Bruton, Gus Cairns, Michael Carter, Leigh Chislett, Ann Chiswick, Simon Collins, James Crane, Arthur Crow, Hilary Curtis, Norman Fowler, Brian Gazzard, Jonathan Grimshaw, Graham Hart, George Hodson, Annie Hoile, Robert James, Pauline Jelliman, Ruth Lowbury, Jacquie Mok, Mark Nelson, Eileen Nixon, John O'Callaghan, Godwyns Onwuchekwa, Diana Onyango, Nick Partridge, Roy Robertson, Chris Rogers, Lorraine Sherr, Christopher Sandford, Chris Smith, Christopher Spence, David Stuart, Flick Thorley, Tricia Warnes, Simon Watney, Shaun Watson, Rupert Whitaker, Tony Whitehead, Ian Williams, Chris Woolls, and Mike Youle.

We are very grateful to Anna Cheshire for her contributions that included coordinating the research, conducting interviews, securing Ethical Committee approval, and managing the transcripts and data so effectively.

CARA (now River House Trust) provided financial support for the project, and we appreciate their help. The University of Westminster, and the Central North West London NHS Foundation Trust hosted the authors during the project's development and completion.

Jeffrey Weeks gave us much valued encouragement and insights from the very start of the project. Helpful reflections that contributed to shaping the book were provided by those that commented on early drafts: Jeremy Booth, Jane Bruton, Michael Carter, Harry Dickinson, Paul Glynn, Peter Gordon, George Hodson, and David Munns. Luise Pattinson, from The Book House, Thame, Oxon, was most efficient in providing assistance in obtaining copies of hard-to-find books.

Grace McInness, Senior Editor, and Evie Lonsdale and Ruth Anderson, Editorial Assistants, Routledge, gave us support throughout the development and completion stages of the book.

Chapter 7 contains material included in our paper Catalan J, Ridge D, Cheshire A, Hedge B & Rosenfeld D (2020) The Changing Narratives of Death, Dying, and HIV in the UK. *Quality of Life Research*, 30(10), 1561–1571, doi:10.1177/1049732320922510. We are grateful to Anna Cheshire and Dana Rosenfeld for their contributions.

Introduction

In our work with people living with HIV, we realised that, 40 years on, many of those activists and professionals involved throughout this time were now retiring, and that most of those still living with HIV are now ageing and many are facing complex medical problems. We believed that if we did not capture their memories and experiences now, they would be lost forever. We think that, against the current picture of successful treatments, we are at risk of marginalising the stories of creativity and survival but also of suffering, and the key lessons learnt by the individuals and communities affected by HIV. With more reliable ways of preventing the spread of the infection and with effective ways of treating those infected with the virus, could crucial stories and wisdom from the frontline of the epidemic be lost? Furthermore, the evolution of developments generated by the epidemic, such as putting people at the centre of their care, have resulted in wide-ranging consequences beyond HIV itself, which are worth highlighting and continuing to fight for.

In the early 1980s, the UK witnessed an explosion of concern about the HIV and AIDS epidemic, focusing at the beginning on 'risk groups', such as gay men and injecting drug users, and only later on the general population. During the last two decades of the twentieth century, infection fears and the exposure to images of sick and dying people, mostly young men, had a significant impact on attitudes to people living and dying with HIV, and more specifically on the provision of health and social care for them. As progress in the understanding of HIV grew and effective treatments were developed, a certain degree of complacency about HIV started to emerge, associated with a loss of the societal memory about the experiences of those early decades. HIV began to be seen as a problem sorted or, at least, as a problem affecting people in faraway countries.

What started tragically, as Crew starkly put it – "AIDS starts with the deaths. With the dying … later there were tests" (Crewe, 2018, p7), was followed by impressive progress. Advances in the treatment of people with HIV have indeed exceeded early expectations, as was the case with the prevention of its transmission. These advances have had an extraordinary impact not just on survival, but also on quality of life. As a senior HIV physician who was involved in care and research from the early days said: "I now believe in miracles". In spite of such progress, health and social difficulties have not disappeared, nor has stigma simply melted away. As an activist living with HIV put it:

> *And the story of AIDS is obviously the story of enormous achievement but it is also the story of injustices.*

There are many facets and layers to the HIV epidemic and its history, and in the words of Rosenberg (1992, p292), AIDS revealed "the inadequacy of any one-dimensional approach to disease, either the social constructionist or the more conventional mechanistically oriented perspective". In this book, we focus on the experiences and responses of key individuals in terms of the care and support offered to people with HIV, as well as prevention of the spread of the virus. To do this, we have relied on a tried and tested approach in the social sciences, namely qualitative semi-structured interviews and thematic analyses (applying the principles of constant comparison to ensure rigorous conclusions) (Braun and Clarke, 2006; Dye, Schatz, Rosenberg, and Coleman, 2000). We collected and analysed data, and in this book report the meanings people attached to the epidemic, their everyday experiences, and the actions of people living with HIV (PLWH), activists, healthcare workers, charity workers, and politicians. They all lived through the tragedy, disappointments, hope, and progress of the last four decades, and survived to tell their account.

Thus, the contents of this book are the product of the passion of the authors and of their research, where we gathered up and analysed systematically the voices of protagonists from the coalface. Having gained approval from the Psychology Ethics Committee at the University of Westminster (Application ID ETH1617-0452), these voices were recorded digitally, transcribed and entered into NVivo software for analysis by the authors (Bazeley and Jackson, 2013), both individually and jointly to reveal people's experiences and perceptions of the epidemic, their responses to it, and to document and illustrate changes over time. We aimed also to consider the consequences and lessons learnt from the HIV story that might be applicable to other health-related conditions, both today and in the future.

Ours is not a comprehensive history of this complex and dramatic period, but rather a scholarly account of personal stories related to HIV care and prevention in the UK, by people who over the last four decades have found themselves at the forefront of the HIV crisis, and have struggled in various ways to get through it and contain its worst effects. Their accounts illustrate Jenkins' view that "History is the way people(s) create, in part, their identities" (Jenkins, 1991, p19). They are, therefore, best placed to shed light on the drama, setbacks, hopes, and progress. Their efforts to provide human relief and succour to people living with HIV reveal the very best of human nature. Their struggles to resist the darker forces of stigma and discrimination, while providing care and vision, changed the social and political outlook of the HIV epidemic – and health care – for the better. We hope their accounts will contribute to validating the experiences of those who faced the HIV pandemic globally, as well as inspire those who face the latest and future viral pandemics. In turn, we expect and hope that these narratives will stir future generations of activists, practitioners, and people living with other health conditions.

Who are the participants? We have included people from a wide range of backgrounds who have played a significant role in the HIV epidemic in the UK, both those who reflect the demographics of the epidemic, and those involved in providing care and support to people living with HIV (PLWH). We recognise the relatively small number of women's voices represented here, a situation well known in many areas of everyday life and in medicine (Criado-Perez, 2019), and similarly the limited number from ethnic minorities. About a third of the participants are women, and one in ten from ethnic minorities. Forty per cent are PLWH, including men that have sex with men (MSM), men with haemophilia, injecting drug users (IDU), and those who acquired HIV through heterosexual sex. Healthcare workers, including doctors and nurses, represent 45% of the participants, and academics, politicians, clergy, and policy makers also contributed their narratives. While many participants are London-based, we interviewed participants from other parts of the UK, including Edinburgh, Manchester, Liverpool, and Brighton. The socio-demographic details of our participants are summarised in the Appendix. While participants' individual responses are anonymised, we show our appreciation for their contributions by including a list of those involved in our Acknowledgements.

The book has two sections. Part I describes the epidemic through accounts of those who were involved during successive historical periods of the development and progress of the epidemic in the UK from 1981, when the first case of AIDS was reported, to the end of the second decade of the twenty-first century, when major progress in treatment of HIV and prevention of its transmission had taken place. These four decades present dramatic changes in the extent of the epidemic, in the individual and social responses to it, and the understanding of its medical and social impact.

In Part II, we focus on some of the lessons that can be learnt and the legacy of the HIV epidemic, including developments in the provision of care and prevention of HIV, the changing narratives about death and dying, and changes in social attitudes to HIV and sexuality. We hope that the lessons learnt from the care and prevention of the HIV epidemic will also be relevant in the future for the management of other viral pandemics, such as COVID-19 (Gorna, 2020; Hargreaves and Davey, 2020).

Who are we, the authors of the book? Two of us (JC and BH) have worked in the UK as frontline mental health clinicians and academic researchers from the start of the epidemic until the second decade of the twenty-first century, and the third (DR) was active in HIV prevention efforts in Australia from the 1980s, as well as being a scholar investigating the social and psychological aspects of HIV, and a psychotherapist in practice working with the epidemic. The words of Svetlana Alexievich (2005, p235) in her oral history of the Chernobyl disaster, best resonate with us even after all these years: "I used to travel among other people's suffering, but here I am as much a witness as the others. My life is part of this event. I live here, with all of this."

While we three are the authors, it is to the participants, with their own voices, we hope to have done justice. They describe their feelings, perspectives, and experiences, which have given shape and direction to the book. They have reminded us all before we forget, of the tragedies, struggles, achievements, lessons, and further opportunities as well as challenges facing us.

References

Alexievich S (2005) *Voices from Chernobyl: the oral history of a nuclear disaster.* New York, Picador.

Bazeley P and Jackson K (2013) *Qualitative data analysis with NVivo.* London, Sage Publications.

Braun V and Clarke V (2006) Using thematic analysis in psychology. *Qualitative Research in Psychology,* 3(2), 77–101. doi:10.1191/1478088706qp063oa

Crewe T (2018) Here was plague. *The London Review of Books,* 40(18), 7–12.

Criado-Perez C (2019) *Invisible women: exposing data bias in a world designed for men.* London, Chatto & Windus.

Dye JI, Schatz IM, Rosenberg BA, and Coleman ST (2000) Constant comparison method: a kaleidoscope of data. *The Qualitative Report,* 4(1/2), 1–10, https://nsuworks.nova.edu/tqr/vol4/iss1/8/

Gorna R (2020) Lessons of Aids for Covid-19: don't sacrifice science to expediency. *Maverick Citizen* Op-Ed, 9 April 2020, https://www.dailymaverick.co.za/author/robin-gorna/

Hargreaves J and Davey C (2020) Three lessons for the COVID-19 response from pandemic HIV. *The Lancet HIV,* 13 April 2020. https://doi.org/10.1016/S2352-3018(20)30110-7

Jenkins, K (1991) *Re-thinking history.* London, Routledge.

Rosenberg CE (1992) *Explaining epidemics and other studies in the history of medicine.* Cambridge, Cambridge University Press.

Part I

Setting the scene: The chronology of HIV hope and despair

1   The dawning of the HIV epidemic

Introduction

The HIV epidemic in the UK was foretold by alarming news of a health crisis developing in the US, accompanied by sensationalist reports in the media about a new disease. This condition initially appeared to affect men that had sex with men (MSM), injecting drug users (IDU), and recipients of blood products. While at first the disease was perceived as a problem only occurring in the US, the threat soon appeared to be closing in on the UK. In what has been called 'the period of moral panic' (Weeks, 2018, p323), the media wasted little time in apportioning guilt to some and absolution to others: people with haemophilia were described by the Daily Express newspaper as the 'AIDS innocents', while gay men and drug users by extension were deserving of their illness (Crewe, 2018).

The first official report about what came to be known as AIDS (Acquired Immune Deficiency Syndrome) was published in June of 1981 in the US by the Centers for Disease Control (CDC, 1981) describing five cases of Pneumocystis Carinii Pneumonia (PCP) in previously healthy young gay men in Los Angeles, and the UK followed later that year with a report of the death of a previously healthy young gay man (DuBois, Branthwaite, Mikhail, and Batten, 1981). Gay-related immune deficiency (GRID) was an early name for this syndrome, later replaced by AIDS. Speculation about its cause, including the possible role of recreational use of amyl nitrate (poppers), was finally settled when in 1983 the virus linked to the syndrome was identified (Barre-Sinoussi, Chermann, Nugeyre, Chamaret et al, 1983), named initially Human T-cell lymphotropic virus type III (HTLV-III) and Lymphadenopathy-associated virus (LAV), and later Human Immunodeficiency Virus (HIV). In 1984 tests were developed to screen for the virus, and by 1985 the first ELISA tests to detect HIV antibodies became available worldwide.

Between 1981 and 1985, gay men were the main group affected, and a gradually developing awareness of the condition led to the communities affected by AIDS to start forming voluntary organisations, such as the Terrence Higgins Trust (THT) in 1983 (Garfield, 1994, p38; Weeks, 2018, p323). These community organisations initially emerged from the gay liberation movements of the 1970s, which had created organisations such as the Gay Liberation Front (GLF), the Campaign for Homosexual Equality, Gay Switchboard, and Friend, which combined political action, law reform, and the provision of counselling and support (Weeks, 2016, p185–230). In what has been termed 'policy from below' (Berridge, 1996, p13–36), gay activists, clinicians, and researchers developed informal links and coordinated action at a time when governments in the UK and the US showed little interest (France, 2016, p13–43; Hallsor, 2017).

The first cases of HIV in people with haemophilia in the UK were diagnosed in 1983. It soon became clear that the infection was linked to a self-administered concentrate of the clotting agent Factor VIII that was introduced in the early 1970s, most of it imported from the US (Garfield, 1994, p60–91). In Edinburgh, a high proportion of injecting drug users were found to be HIV positive in the mid-1980s (Robertson, Bucknall, Welsby, Roberts et al, 1986), and this followed an outbreak of hepatitis B that spread rapidly among them. Their stored blood revealed that most had HIV. As an HIV physician said at the time:

> *It isn't going to be if HIV comes, it is to be when it comes.*

Injecting heroin, and sharing injecting equipment due to difficulties accessing sterile needles and syringes, contributed to the development of the epidemic. Local police were particularly active confiscating injecting equipment, increasing the likelihood of sharing. Even on the hospital wards needles used to take blood had to be locked up to stop patients' visitors from taking them away and reusing them (Garfield, 1994, p92–105). A psychiatric nurse commented:

> *One of my patients came back to the city and was present at one of the shooting galleries that were prevalent at the time, cleaning the needles in a pot of dirty water in the middle of a table.*

From gay liberation to HIV charities

Against a background of increasing alarm and uncertainty, activists schooled in the battles of early gay liberation started to organise and develop links with clinicians, partly to provide support to those affected by the new disease or worried about its personal impact, as well as to help educate, and fight discrimination. A shift of priorities and objectives among those already engaged in voluntary community action, even when not always centred on gay issues, provided the basis for the early HIV community organisations. Usually, proximity to somebody who had become ill or died with HIV provided the stimulus for action. This account by one of the early activists points to the birth of the Terrence Higgins Trust (THT), a charity that started as the Terry Higgins Trust to raise funding for research, and later broadened its role to include education and support, and that eventually played a key role in better managing the epidemic in the UK. What is striking in this account is the combination of powerful emotion and commitment, and clear practical thinking:

> *After university I started working with the Gay Switchboard as a volunteer, and that was when the first reports of a new disease started coming. The press in general ignored it, apart from the odd sensationalist report, but the gay press was reporting it. The Gay*

Switchboard together with the Health Education Council invited a speaker from the New York Gay Men's Health Crisis, and there some London doctors too, friends of Terry Higgins, whose name had got into the gay press as the first identified person to have died [4th July 1982]. I was in the audience and I was viscerally moved. At the end of the meeting I got up and said to the hall, the Switchboard is dealing with so many calls from worried gay people, and I think we need to support the friends of Terry Higgins who had set up a trust in his name, and raise money. So, we then developed the THT charity, we knew it had to be expanded, raising money and giving information, and we broadened the remit somewhat by bringing a lot more education.

As news of the growing number of people becoming ill and dying spread, many were fearful and did not know where to turn. THT set up an essential helpline providing a source where the latest accurate information could be provided. In the absence of any real understanding of the disease, its causes, means of transmission, and treatment, dealing with the fear of becoming unwell and what at the time seemed inevitable death for those affected became critical.

This led early on to the development of community-based services to support people in such critical states of fear and disease. For some time, HIV-positive gay men in THT had provided mutual support, meeting informally to talk about their health, treatment, and for pointers about how to cope with HIV-related problems. These self-selected 'new families' were replacing biological families when their support was lacking. A new group, Body Positive, developed local support throughout the country. This was in parallel with efforts to provide suitable forms of professional care, despite only a gradual emergence of knowledge about the condition itself. Early initiatives to provide counselling for people living and dying with HIV illustrate how personal experiences and relationships were key to the early organic development of HIV services. Here, the scale and urgency of the many needs facing people living with HIV (PLWH) were becoming increasingly apparent. An HIV charity worker described the early stages of development of a community-based organisation:

I was freelance and partly working as a counsellor, but with a special interest in death and dying, and bereavement and loss. And because of that I was often working with people with life threatening illnesses. I had started a little counselling centre in the base- ment of our own house, where I did workshops and classes in death and dying. And by the time a close friend died and a nurse from the local hospital attended a workshop, I realised that something was very wrong and we need to tackle it quickly. I was then approached by Body Positive, and we started doing courses for people living with HIV. I remember that we used to do open meetings, and I remember one when the basement was full to overflowing and there were people outside listening through the window. Suddenly this thing was happening and large numbers of people were emerging, and that was how I learned just what the social climate was, and what people were up against in terms of employment, housing, and accessing healthcare.

As in the case of the development of the THT, awareness of what was going on around them led volunteers, who were already providing support and counselling for people facing severe illness, to focus on the dawning HIV epidemic and form new community-based organisations.

One of the issues that surfaced at the time was the scope of work covered by the charities. For example, the THT debated whether they should just provide direct services to PLWH or whether they should have a wider remit, such as lobbying government to provide statutory services. The charity volunteers had no experience of lobbying, policy making, or of advising on ways to stay safe from HIV. So, a diversity of approaches was adopted culminating later in 1985 in an alliance between the Medical, and the Health Promotion Groups of the THT and doctors and nurses. Together they pulled together the first safer sex guidelines, 'Facts about AIDS' and 'More Facts about AIDS for Gay Men'. These became influential publications, even though some gay men considered them anti-sex propaganda (Callen, 1989; Garfield and Davenport-Hines, 1995).

The beginnings of a person-centred model of care

Early on, a trickle of people with HIV were referred to hospitals, but they tended to concentrate in centres that had a reputation for good care and non-discriminatory practice. Eventually, a loose network of clinics and wards with an interest in treating people with HIV emerged. The novelty of the disease, the challenges of caring for very sick people, the high death rates, and the intense stigmatisation of people living with HIV (PLWH) in the media and in the public discourse, helped to create an alliance between a community of committed activists and sympathetic professionals, who talked to each other, shared information, and took action. Soon, innovative approaches were emerging in the face of increasing pressures on these HIV-related services. For instance, insistence on the involvement of PLWH in their own care became an early feature of clinical services. In the face of hostile wider politics, somehow this alliance was able to achieve a kind of care that had never been seen to any large extent in the NHS before. An activist living with HIV recalls those early days:

> There was no HIV and then there was HIV. It came from nothing and then there were horrific times of discrimination, and it was very nasty. The context in the '80s was very divisive politics ... and you had a few doctors, who tended to be young and who were from different disciplines that included GU medicine, who actually saw beyond what was happening and how impossible as a medical problem this new condition was. And they slowly built specialised services that were able to provide some reasonable shelter from the nightmare that was going on outside. In the US, gay doctors from the communities that were affected helped to establish the first services by developing HIV exclusive clinics, and with that approaches to care changed, and very early on you had the concept that people who were directly affected had to be involved in their care, and you had similar units developing in the UK.

The commitment of NHS health worker teams to provide good care was remarked upon by many of our participants, even as they acknowledged that understanding of the disease was back then very limited. With committed staff but no effective treatments, care gravitated towards being centred on the particular needs of patients coming through the door. Thus, listening to PLWH and creating an alliance with them made sense, as one PLWH recalls:

> *A friend of ours came back from San Francisco in 1981 and commented that there it was like watching skeletons push trolleys around in the supermarket. It was quite scary, nobody knew what was going on, but at the same time my partner was getting quite ill … He lost weight, had dysentery, I don't think the KS had started by then. So, it was about '82 that the doctors said, look we think it's HTLV-3, and he spent a long time in hospital that year. The care was fantastic, but it was only treating symptomatic things. We had huge support from the doctors. Everything was observational, everything relied on what the patient told you, not vice versa. Still nowadays HIV care is the gold standard for the NHS because that has never been lost. People had to work together, although nobody knew what was going on, the interest in caring was amazing.*

Unlike other PLWH, patients with haemophilia attending Haemophilia Centres tended to have pre-established, close, and longstanding relationships with their doctors and nurses. As the HIV epidemic developed, and it became clear that they had been infected, concerns about the future of this group of patients grew. In a similar way to the case of other groups of people affected by HIV, clinical teams here also maintained their support for patients, even if there was little clarity about what to do. A man with haemophilia and HIV remembers the confusion and uncertainty of the time:

> *We thought we were going to die very quickly. Now that's not to say we hadn't been reassured, definitely the day we were given the test results and, repeatedly every time we saw the doctors afterwards, which was probably as frequent as once a month. They were saying that the virus may have a role in this disease, that's not proved, and it may be that only a small proportion of people with the virus go on to develop this disease. They were full of optimism and hope, although any of the practical questions I could think of to ask them, the answer was always, we don't know. But they nevertheless had sensible, practical basic infection control which worked for us.*

Early interest in HIV from doctors and care professionals

Early on, specialised outpatient and inpatient services – needed to cope with ever increasing numbers of patients – started to become established in the early '80s. This was around the time when a generation of doctors and nurses with a keen interest in HIV began to emerge on the scene. In many instances this was the start of a lifetime commitment, and a number of these professionals continue to work in the field today, although others have reached retirement age. A variety of factors led to the attraction to this medical specialty. Gay doctors, who might have known many PLWH in their private lives, had an obvious interest in HIV, and recognised the impending crisis:

> *At first, I met people with HIV through my involvement in gay community organisations, and later through social networks, when close friends became ill. At the time, it was*

very difficult to be open about it, and it was spoken about in hushed tones. The enormity of what seemed to be happening gave a sense of urgency to the need to do something.

There was also the intellectual challenge of coping with a dramatically new disease of unknown aetiology with complex manifestations and the expectation of poor outcome. As one doctor intimated, the excitement and appeal of working in this new pioneering area drew people in, and made it a difficult field to leave:

I got a research job at the STD clinic working on herpes viruses and their treatment, and I was training to become an obstetrician and gynaecologist. One of the clinics had developed an interest in HIV Persistent Generalised Lymphadenopathy, and there was a PGL clinic with research fellows, and I ended up spending two years there. I had wanted to do Obs and Gynae, but I changed plans, and the driving force was the amazing ignorance that we had about AIDS and HIV, [and] the energy that people were putting in to try and cure that ignorance both scientifically and in terms of public perception and stigma, [and this] was something I wanted to be part of. The HIV clinic was the most exciting place to work in the hospital. It drew people from all sorts of other fields of training, nobody was a straightforward physician, and nobody was trained in what we had to do.

As PLWH tended to belong to stigmatised populations, this added an especially human and political dimension that attracted care professionals searching for something different, or who had a social conscience. At the same time, patients with HIV and their doctors tended to be of similar age and background, and this also fostered connection and empathy, as an HIV physician remembers:

I was doing research on cancer, and in 1979 I saw my first HIV [patient], although I didn't know it at the time, he had all sort of things wrong with him, and we knew that he had no T4 cells but we didn't know why. Then in 1981 my senior registrar was in San Francisco and wrote to me and said, there is a new disease sweeping the States, which is presenting with Pneumocystis Carinii Pneumonia [PCP]. And I always quite liked rare diseases, so I read about it and thought, well, that's interesting. And that very same week a patient presented with a chest X-ray of PCP, me having just literally read about it all. So, I sat in the X-ray conference and said very confidently, oh, that's PCP and he must have some Pentamidine. Nobody else had heard of it, of course and they all thought 1) that I was wrong, and then 2) subsequently, which is also a lie, that I was near genius. That is how it started for me. I knew virtually nothing about gay men then, I was about 35 years old, and a whole new world opened to me, of different relationships, of different ways of people thinking and different activities, and what they were doing with their lives.

For some doctors, their interest had started when they were still at medical school. Sometimes this interest developed for very personal reasons, especially, but not always, if students were lesbian, gay, bisexual, or trans (LGBTQ) themselves. A doctor recalls life as a gay medical student:

The first time I heard about HIV was not about HIV but about Kaposi's sarcoma, while reading a gay magazine in 1980 or '81 … I also remember people developing illnesses, at the time thought to be 'glandular fever', and of course that was their seroconversion, but nobody knew what it was. We are talking about pre-internet days. So, what was happening was that people were reporting things, the first papers came out in 1981. In 1982 I was in my fourth year at medical school, and I wrote a dissertation on 'What is the aetiology of Gay-Related Immune Deficiency (GRID)?' and I read everything that had been written in one afternoon in the library, and there in total six, seven papers, that was all there was to go on. When it came to my final exams, there was a question about GRID, and I found out later I was the only person in the medical school who had answered that particular question. I was the first openly gay medical student there, and apart from me, very few people were interested in the topic.

Such was the compelling and public nature of the condition that for some, early interest and concern about a new disease that started to develop while at medical school came to fruition later, even when their teachers at the time had not shared their curiosity:

I first heard about HIV as a medical student, and I can remember because it was something new and something a bit strange. I remember we were doing community medicine, and we had to write an essay on the epidemiology of syphilis or an alternative subject, and I said I wanted to do it on HIV, but the professor said, well that's a nothing disease, and we all had to do the essay on syphilis. When I qualified and was doing house jobs I came across many sick patients with HIV, and after doing some general medicine I came back to the HIV ward.

Doctors working with injecting drug users faced particular difficulties in relation to prescribing opiates for HIV-related conditions, or simply in managing their drug dependence, given the stigma attached to drug users and, in some areas, the epidemic nature of drug problems. Despite the problems that such doctors were up against in working in the area, including the large scale of the problem, these obstacles seemed to have been a challenge worth pursuing for the individuals concerned. An experienced general practitioner and academic remembers the tensions and concerns of those early days:

… the first thing I remember is reading in the Sunday paper about GRID in gay men in California, and then I remember somebody who had been a fellow student at university and was now working in New York telling me about drug users and shooting galleries there. It resonated with me because we had a big problem in the city. As a trainee GP I had seen heroin users admitted to hospital who became agitated and were injecting drugs on the ward. My consultant advised me to prescribe heroin and that controlled prescribing helped her while she was there. When I became a GP, we had loads of young kids, whole loads of people injecting heroin, whole generations of kids leaving the local schools at the same time and injecting heroin. It was just like Irvine Welsh described it in 'Trainspotting'. There was an epidemic of heroin use. It was quite shocking.

Nurses working on the ward, in outpatient clinics, and in the community, soon also acquired a prominent role in the care of PLWH. As in the case of doctors, nurses felt drawn by the terrible predicament faced by their patients, being both highly stigmatised in the wider community, and also seriously ill. However, in the very early days, such empathy was not always possible to translate into good care given the fear among colleagues, as an HIV nurse remarked:

> *I was training to be a nurse, and a close friend of mine's friend was diagnosed with HTLV-III as it was then called, and he died. Later we had a patient in the psychiatric ward with HTLV-III, and he was the first patient I looked after with it, and it was pretty hideous because he was severely mentally ill and really disturbed and been treated appallingly by the health system – we had to isolate him, we were all covered in plastic and double gloved, even his notes were covered in plastic, all his bedding was thrown away and burnt, everything he touched was thrown away.*

Nurses reported that they tried their best to provide support and care. In the end, nurses said they developed strong and empathetic relationships with their patients. Some were LGBTQ themselves, and so had known a few of the PLWH they were caring for in their private lives. One such male nurse described his feelings and productive reaction:

> *I was in a gay pub, I was about 18 or 19, and somebody said, have you heard about that gay men thing in America, this weird cancer thing, and there was this hushed silence. I remember being really impacted by what they were saying, and this older guy he went, don't worry, it's an American thing, it will never come here. I think everybody wanted to believe that but we knew. And then there was a programme on TV, 'Killer in the Village', a documentary, and when you look at it now, it looks like a wildlife programme, because it's that, 'these are homosexuals'. I remember watching it at home and being really impacted by and intrigued by what was going on. I think I have always hated injustice, and there was a lot of bad press and bigotry and cruelty in the attitudes to what was happening, and I think that really fired me up. I then came to London to do my nursing training, and then went to work in a sexual health clinic.*

He was not alone in his response. Other nurses also had a strong sense of social justice and commitment, and so were open to understanding their patients within a wider context and with the aim of addressing injustice and stigma towards PLWH:

> *I trained between '78 and '81 and worked in general medicine. I had been political as a student, involved in the early days of the women's movement and gay rights, so I was politically aware, and in those days, there was also a miners' strike, and I was very involved. I hadn't come across HIV patients in my general ward yet, but I was really interested in whether I could get the opportunity to work with them, because the press was so awful about what was happening, and having been involved in the various movements about human rights, I wanted to be there, I wanted to do something about it, basically.*

The psychological impact of HIV was recognised from the start of the epidemic, and psychologists, psychiatric nurses, and to a lesser degree, psychiatrists, started to explore their new roles in the context of HIV. A clinical psychologist described her early interest in HIV infection:

> *I heard about HIV when I was training to be a clinical psychologist, and I was already an academic, and in one of my placements there was a gay psychologist whose boyfriend was sick, and I think he started telling me that they were waiting for tests to come from the US, and I became quite interested, and this psychologist informed me, and helped me develop an interest.*

A psychiatric nurse working with drug users with HIV infection described her move from neuropsychological research to a clinical role in response to the stories and problems outlined by her patients:

> *The work doing brain research was interesting, but actually it was the patients that attracted me to the job. They had such a raw deal in life, so many of them were born in pretty horrible circumstances, they came from the grottiest areas of the city, some of them had had no parenting. Their parents were often alcoholics, because that was the sort of drug addiction in their parents' generation, and some of them were also drug users. I remember one married couple who had both grown up in a religious children's home, and they told stories of having to share a bed, and you took it in turns to be on the outside of the bed, because the person on the outside of the bed would be abused by the monks that night. Was it any wonder that they grew up addicted to substances that made them feel better? So, I got to know them extremely well, and that was very helpful when it came to developing their drug regimens.*

As in the case of physicians and nurses, some LGBTQ mental health workers had experience of working in community organisations involved in fighting for LGBTQ rights that made them aware of the psychological distress and stigma faced by PLWH. Again, interest further developed when HIV impacted on their personal networks, as described by a psychiatrist:

> *I became aware of HIV in about '82 or '83, partly through the gay press and reports from the US about this new disease, GRID. I had been involved in Friend, the gay and lesbian counselling group, and we were beginning to get callers concerned about the news. I was doing a psychiatric placement at the local STD clinic, where there was a good deal of interest in psychological and sexual problems. I just happened to be in the place where people were being referred and where health advisors started to develop new skills to support people who were becoming ill or were worried about developing a serious illness. I vividly remember my first patient, and have often wondered what happened to her. As a gay man, HIV seemed a very important issue to get to grips with, and I quickly recognised its likely mental health consequences.*

Are we ready for what is coming?

The start of the epidemic in the UK in 1981 reflected some of the developments seen in the US, with an early involvement of the communities affected by HIV infection. The courage and commitment of individuals with a track record of involvement in community organisations concerned with LGBTQ rights was fundamental in the emergence of HIV-related campaigning and support charities and organisations, at a time when government bodies had not woken up to the developing crisis. In parallel with these early responses, healthcare workers dealing with PLWH being referred to the hospital services, started to respond to the needs of their patients by developing models of care that directly involved their patients in dealing with a disease that, at the time, was not well understood, had no effective treatment, and had very poor outcome, against a background of stigma and rejection of PLWH.

The foundations for the beginning of a coordinated response to HIV infection were established in these early attempts to understand, reach out, and provide support. It was not entirely clear at that stage what the tragic impact of the developing epidemic would be, and how it would affect so many lives, as discussed in the next chapter.

References

Barre-Sinoussi F, Chermann JC, Nugeyre MT, Chamaret S, Gruest J, Dauget C, Axler-Blin C, Vezinet-Brun F, Rouzioux C, Rozenbaum W, and Montagnier L (1983) Isolation of a T-lymphotropic retrovirus from a patient at risk for AIDS. *Science*, 220(4599), 868–871.

Berridge V (1996) *AIDS in the UK: the making of policy, 1981–1994*. Oxford, Oxford University Press.

Callen M (1989) In defence of anal sex. *PWA Coalition Newsline*, 41, 37–43.

CDC (1981) Pneumocystis carinii pneumonia – Los Angeles. *Mortality and Morbidity Weekly Report*, 30, 250–252.

Crewe T (2018) Here was plague. *The London Review of Books*, 40(18), 7–16.

DuBois RM, Branthwaite MA, Mikhail JR, and Batten JC (1981) Primary Pneumocystis carinii and Cytomegalovirus infections. *The Lancet*, 2, 1339.

France D (2016) *How to survive a plague: the story of how activists and scientists tamed AIDS*. London, Picador.

Garfield S (1994) *The end of innocence: Britain in the time of AIDS*. London, Faber and Faber.

Garfield S and Davenport-Hines R (1995) The end of innocence: Britain in the time of AIDS. *Nature*, 373(6509), 29.

Hallsor S (2017) A comparison of early responses to AIDS in the UK and the US. *RES MEDICA, Journal of the Royal Medical Society*, 24(1), 57–64. doi:10.2218/resmedica. v24i1.1558

Robertson JR, Bucknall A, Welsby P, Roberts J, Inglis J, Peutherer J, and Brettle R (1986) Epidemic of AIDS related virus (HTLV-III/LAV) infection among intravenous drug users. *British Medical Journal*, 292, 527–529. doi:10.1136/bmj.292.6519.527

Weeks J (2016) *Coming out: the emergence of LGBT identities from the 19th century to the present* (4th edn). London, Quartet Books Ltd.

Weeks J (2018) *Sex, politics and society: the regulation of sexuality since 1800* (4th edn). London, Routledge.

2 The horror

Introduction

The years 1985–1987 ushered in a worldwide AIDS epidemic with devastating consequences. This prompted both national and international actions, with the World Health Organisation (WHO) holding the first International AIDS conference in Atlanta, Georgia. The extensive media coverage of the death of Rock Hudson from AIDS in 1985 gave widespread attention to the illness, just as testing for Human T-cell lymphotropic virus type III (HTLV-III) became available in many clinics across the UK. Fearing the impact a positive test result might have, the Department of Health and Social Security (DHSS) guidelines required counselling to be provided at testing sites (DHSS, 1985). The following year the International Committee on the Taxonomy of Viruses agreed on naming the virus 'Human Immuno-deficiency Virus' (HIV).

The UK government, recognising the crisis, formed the AIDS Cabinet committee and ran a newspaper campaign in an attempt to disseminate information about the risks of infection. At this time too came evidence that HIV could be spread from an infected mother to her unborn child, with the first baby with HIV in the UK recorded in Lothian in 1986. The Royal College of Obstetricians and Gynaecologists issued guidelines on pregnancy (Royal College of Obstetricians and Gynaecologists, 1987) that stressed the serious risks of vertical transmission, and strongly advised women with HIV not to get pregnant. With mounting concern in government, on 21 November 1986 Norman Fowler, the Secretary of State for Health, in an emergency debate in the House of Commons, announced £20 million for a public health campaign to limit the spread of infection.

Early in 1987 Norman Fowler, during an international fact-finding tour, was at once impressed and moved by the community-based model of care he found operating in San Francisco. On return to the UK he extended funding from that already allocated to basic scientific research and education and prevention measures, to that for the direct care of people living with HIV (PLWH). Funds rose from an allocation of £680,000 in 1985–1986 to £2.5 million in the year 1986–1987. From this funding came innovations such as the new, dedicated AIDS ward at the Middlesex Hospital, which was opened in April 1987 by Princess Diana.

With money now being made available for the care of PLWH both through the healthcare services and the voluntary sector, the government made attempts, initially through the AIDS Control Act (1987), to coordinate and monitor the various providers. After a number of failed attempts, with providers vying for leadership, in 1987 the DHSS funded the National AIDS Trust (NAT) to coordinate the HIV-related voluntary sector, and the National AIDS helpline, a telephone counselling service. Many volunteers from the gay support helplines, with no other income, took the opportunity to be paid for their input and with less available voluntary support not all helplines managed to survive. A national centre, the National AIDS Counselling Training Unit (NACTU) was set up to train counsellors in the specific issues facing those at risk or diagnosed with HIV. The year 1987 also saw attempts to provide education and prevention messages to the public with the UK government 'Don't Die of Ignorance' campaign and 'AIDS week'; a week of TV, radio, and poster campaigns and discussions.

As increasing numbers of gay men were being diagnosed with AIDS and dying, in 1987 an influential political direct-action group in New York, ACT UP (the AIDS Coalition to Unleash Power), formed to confront authorities and demand action to protect those at risk and those infected with HIV. In the UK the needs of those dying with AIDS-related illnesses were met by the opening of two hospices, the Mildmay Mission Hospital in Shoreditch and the London Lighthouse in West London. Internationally, the extent and gravity of the rising epidemic led the WHO to declare 1 December 1988 the first World AIDS Day.

The horror: HIV has arrived

Testing

By 1985 a reliable test for the presence of antibodies to the virus HTLV-III (later to be known as HIV) became widely available in sexual health clinics. But with no cure for HIV, many at risk wondered whether there was any point to having a test. They faced a dilemma – on the one hand to test and live with the consequences, and on the other, to spend their days constantly worrying whether they were infected, or denying the possibility. People made different decisions about this momentous issue. The DHSS guidelines (DHSS, 1985) required counselling to be available wherever HIV testing was carried out so clinics provided pre- and post-test counselling – first to prepare people, and then to help them process the shock of a positive test result as was appreciated by this gay activist, living with HIV:

> *There was always counselling … because people didn't know how long it would be between infection and frank expression of disease … we were pretty sure that disease meant death.*

In those days, results took up to two weeks to come back – time to imagine the worst while hoping for a reprieve. This could be a terrifying time for those testing: some people never returned for their results. Gay men, especially those who had spent time in the US with friends and partners who were ill or who had died, had developed suspicions that they too might be infected. As one gay man who had tested positive said, for many of us, taking the test and returning a positive result seemed inevitable as we suffered symptoms that were unusual in fit and previously healthy young gay men:

> So, it was Thursday 30th May. It's emblazoned on my memory … And I knew from the symptoms I had; all the lymph nodes in my neck had come up, and they were like bullets … and I had oral thrush and all … I was very calm, because I'd expected it … and I'd prepared myself for it. And I knew … in the back of my mind over those ten days, what [the test result] was going to be.

Even so, hearing the words confirming a positive result was frequently devastating, regardless of how prepared people felt. Many older gay men who had lived through the times when homosexual acts were criminal offences, had married in order to conceal their sexual preferences, but had continued to have sex with men. Now they found themselves infected, and faced telling their wives, not only that they had HIV, but that they also had sex with men.

The haemophilia clinics had little experience of imparting devastating health information. Some patients were not informed of their positive status for years. Others were told during a routine visit to the haemophilia clinic where they came totally unprepared, sometimes with their children, and maybe with no one to support them. The manner in which people with haemophilia were informed of their infection was frequently inadequate and sometimes inaccurate information was given. An activist who had acquired HIV through Factor VIII described his experience:

> And the doctor went through what it might mean. I'd got antibodies to HTLV-3; it could mean that I was immune to it.

It was common for testing in this environment to be undertaken without counselling or consent and results to be given with a lack of sensitivity, as two people with haemophilia remembered:

> My brother and I were told together … And the doctor said we've had the results back and they're positive, and my brother said, Oh God, What a relief.

> Confidentiality wasn't very good. The haemophiliacs with HIV had 'Haemophilia' written on their files in big red letters. For those without – no red letters.

Living with HIV

At the time, with the knowledge that there was no treatment for HIV, a positive result meant that all diagnosed people would face an early death, and a nurse recalls a typical response:

> The effect is so devastating … You know AIDS kills people so this is going to kill you … and if you have sex with someone, it will kill them too.

For some the positive result came as especially traumatising. A Black African woman described her reaction to a positive test result:

> *It's a complete shock for me. I didn't know whether to cry … I was just numb for a long time. After the cups of tea and blah, blah, blah I went on the bus, the right bus, but went all the way [to the end of the route] before I snapped out of it.*

Over the weekend most support agencies shut down. Thus, receiving a positive diagnosis on a Friday meant no help was available until the following Monday. If people had no friends or family to tell, or were scared to do so, they might be alone with their thoughts. Reports of drunken weekends and suicide attempts following HIV-positive results were not uncommon. A moving article in the *British Medical Journal* (Richards, 1986) alerted physicians to the issue and many testing clinics adopted a 'Never on a Friday' approach.

Public attitudes to HIV were largely formed by media reports that were generally aimed at stoking fear, and rarely acceptance of those with the virus. There were instances of ill people being asked to get out of ambulances and walk to A&E. Although there were accounts of gay bashings, non-contact attacks such as excreta though the letterboxes of people suspected of having HIV, of offensive graffiti daubed on their houses, and bricks through windows, were also reported. Consequently, post-test counselling recommendations were that an HIV-positive result should only be revealed to those who could be trusted not to divulge this sensitive information (Miller and Carne, 1987). This strategy was protective but could also result in people largely coping with infection and illness on their own.

When people disclosed their HIV status it could change the way they were seen by friends and colleagues, but as an HIV-positive heterosexual man reflected, there was no way of escaping the ramifications of a HIV-positive result for those with the diagnosis themselves:

> *Whatever others would think of me if they knew, it was as nothing compared with the way I feel about myself.*

For gay men infection was usually directly linked to their sexual behaviours, specifically unprotected anal sex. The guilty versus innocent narrative of HIV at the time led some gay men to question whether the media was correct – was this terrible thing a punishment for being a homosexual? A gay nurse remembers how many felt shame:

> *Some patients [thought] everything people had said about them was true, you got this because you're dirty … well what did [you] expect.*

HIV infected people of all ages, but the majority of those with the infection were young, and they mourned for futures they would never have. However, some managed to be more philosophical about their HIV than others, as the experience of a gay professional diagnosed with HIV illustrates:

> *I thought I was going to die in 6 months, and it gives you a different perspective on life … My doctor said you have to learn to live with uncertainty. And actually, that's not a bad lesson for life, with or without HIV.*

Although by the late 1980s the test for HIV had been widely available for a number of years, with still no reliable treatments, most people didn't get tested until they were sick. By 1986, however, there was a sudden increase in those presenting to hospital sick and dying. Clearly, HIV was not going to be confined to the US as predicted by some; it had already arrived in the UK. Not having been tested, and with little knowledge of the manifestations of infection, people often presented to the hospital with their first AIDS-related illnesses expecting some other, less severe diagnosis. One gay man remembers his shock:

> *I noticed I had a lump in my belly, and I thought it's just a cyst, but I was getting tireder and tireder and it grew … The [doctor] said she thought it was a cancer and it was non-Hodgkin's lymphoma … So I was immediately admitted to an HIV ward … I'd had no preparation for anything HIV … I'd read about it in the papers and had an idea of the facts, but not of the emotions of suddenly being in a ward with 12 people all near death.*

By the end of 1988 over 10,000 people in the UK had tested positive for HIV, with over 2,000 of them (20%) presenting with AIDS, and approximately 1,500 (15%) had died (Public Health England, 2018). A doctor recalled that as the numbers of those infected with HIV grew, medics became increasingly familiar with the presentations of symptomatic HIV infection, conditions not previously linked to young men.

> *They arrived in casualty, and they arrived on the ward bloody sick, and you did a test. You didn't really need to do a test because you knew what it was.*

The doctors at the time knew little more about HIV than did well-informed patients. The underlying infection couldn't be eliminated, and it inevitably led to death. A charity worker described how doctors felt hopeless and impotent against the virus:

> *To have so many young men … becoming very sick, very quickly was a seismic shock particularly to clinicians … They were the first generations who had been trained to cure rather than to care through all the innovations through the 50s, 60s, and 70s.*

As one opportunistic infection was treated, PLWH succumbed to yet another. Although conditions such as Pneumocystis Carinii Pneumonia (PCP), and Cytomegalovirus (CMV) were not themselves new diseases, a doctor described how in PLWH they were very aggressive and could kill:

People got very disabled before they died … disfigured, blind, demented … It wasn't so much that they had cancer and then they died. It's the fact they had multiple different things.

HIV frequently resulted in changes to people's physical appearance such as a dramatic loss of weight or the blackberry coloured skin pigmentations of Kaposi's sarcoma (KS). KS not only openly advertised a positive HIV status but also changed an aspect of self-appearance – that was often of great importance to gay male identity. Such changes were cumulative and eventually took their toll. Many were aware of how near they had come to death. It appeared that it was the cumulative stress of an AIDS diagnosis with multiple fears and concerns being raised simultaneously, that led to a time of acute distress and a collapse in people's ability to cope (Hedge, Petrak, Sherr, Glover, and Slaughter, 1992). Intense reactions such as anxiety, depression, helplessness, hopelessness, guilt, anger, shame, and a loss of self-esteem were commonly experienced, but as a gay man reflected, were not always anticipated:

The physical recovery happened, but the emotional recovery; I was utterly knocked for six … I emotionally collapsed … it manifested as intense anger. I just couldn't cope … I'd been so convinced I was going to die when I was in hospital. I can remember crying, thinking I'm going to die.

The learning curve for clinicians of how HIV could present, and how it could be treated, had to be fast. As the numbers testing positive grew, so too came the realisation that it was not only those with major illnesses who were infected, but that potentially a large number of people were infected but asymptomatic. A picture of a clinical iceberg was emerging. How long the period was between being asymptomatic and being severely ill was not known. Neither, at the time, was it clear whether AIDS was a certain outcome of HIV infection. A doctor working with injecting drug users recalls a conversation with a colleague:

I asked what'll happen to people with HIV and he said probably a percentage of them will develop AIDS and the rest will just get better.

At this time many children and adolescents with haemophilia were not told of their infection as parents feared both their child's response, and public reactions. There was public hysteria over children with HIV in schools with genuine concerns over the way in which schools dealt with cuts, grazes and nose bleeds (*The Times*, 1985). Although the schools themselves quickly adopted universal precautions (i.e. preventing any blood coming into contact with another person), parents frequently continued to object to the presence of HIV-positive children and those who might be, including the children of people with haemophilia in schools. So children were frequently charged with a big secret: they weren't to mention haemophilia outside the house. With the growing awareness that Factor VIII had been contaminated with HIV, some investigated their own HIV status and on finding out that they were positive, they turned to the gay HIV helplines to find answers. With this support some of the inaccurate information such as 'antibodies to HIV could mean you are immune' was corrected. But not all felt comfortable with accessing the voluntary support available that was essentially directed towards gay men.

Those working with viruses had recognised that HIV, a new blood-borne disease found in drug users in New York, would not be confined to the US, as a Scottish doctor stated:

> *It's not going to be if it [HIV] comes; it's going to be when it comes.*

In fact, HIV had already reached drug users in Scotland, long before anyone had realised. In the early 1980s, Edinburgh had experienced a severe outbreak of Hepatitis B that had spread rapidly between drug users. When the blood of drug users stored from this hepatitis outbreak was tested for HIV in 1985 it came as a shock to find that in 1983 approximately 50% were already infected with HIV (Robertson, Bucknall et al., 1986a). It was then realised that infection with HIV was widespread amongst those injecting heroin in Edinburgh and New York, and it became clear that transmission was linked to the sharing of needles and syringes (Robertson et al., 1986a).

With restrictions on the supply of new needles and syringes and many users living in poverty, 'shooting galleries' where equipment was shared (and if cleaned, not adequately), any infection could easily be transmitted. As drug use was not legal, and the lives of many drug users were chaotic, recruitment to studies to accurately estimate the size of the problem across drug-using populations proved difficult. It was unlikely that any could ensure a representative sample of users but the wide differences in prevalence, with Edinburgh at more than 50% (Robertson, Bucknall, and Wiggins, 1986b) and Glasgow and London less than 5%, did suggest that HIV had been introduced at different times, and was dependent on the pattern of mixing of drug users, local drug-injecting practices, and other risk behaviours. But the realisation amongst drug users that they were at risk took time to seep in. HIV was still seen as a gay disease prevalent in the US. In the words of an ex-injecting drug user:

> *We were in a den watching the telly and this guy said … you can get that from jagging, and I said, oh that won't be here. We didn't realise that it was here all along.*

Even before the risk of HIV was appreciated, it was realised that the safest way to inject was to be the first user of equipment. When HIV was discovered, those who were down the line in sharing needles were most vulnerable. As a former injecting drug user understood:

> *My pal … I was using with him, and he always had to have the first stick, and he said I'm HIV, and I said, oh no, no, if you've got it, I've got it.*

The knowledge that HIV could be spread through the transmission of blood as well as through sex was a major concern to health professionals. It meant that there could be no complacency through the assumption that an infection transmitted through gay sex would be confined within the gay population. It became clear that all could become infected through blood. In 1986 the ratio of male to female people infected with HIV in the UK was 33:1 but in Africa the ratio at the time was 1:1 (DHSS, 1987). Here was evidence that HIV could reach the heterosexual population. As fears of the widespread transmission of HIV grew, discussion of 'Risk Groups' moved to the consideration of 'Risk Behaviours' – everyone was now at risk depending on their own specific behaviours.

Responses to the horror

Charity involvement

With the rapid rise in the number of people testing positive for HIV, a plethora of charities were established, each aiming to address the particular needs of specific communities or a specific HIV-related issue. The newly formed charities such as Terrence Higgins Trust (THT), Body Positive, and Crusaid, seeing the difficulties faced by people severely ill and unable to support themselves, fought for the provision of practical daily support. Those who were sick were usually unable to continue with work and, being young, few had savings to see them through hard times. Adequate housing, furniture, and social service interventions were necessary. With limited funds and little energy, PLWH were frequently unable to feed themselves adequately. Charities such as the FOOD Chain coordinated food donations and provided hot meals on Sundays for those who needed it. Perhaps the greatest need was for people who had been abandoned by those close to them to have some personal, reliable support to prevent isolation and loneliness. The Buddy system introduced by THT provided a named volunteer, a Buddy, to befriend a PLWH. Attempts were made to link Buddies with PLWH through demographic data, interests, and personalities. Generally, these matches were successful and Buddies stepped in to provide the input one might expect from a partner, friend, or family member such as visiting when in hospital, accompanying them to the theatre or on shopping trips, or simply being there for tea and a chat in their homes.

Political responses

By 1986, some in government saw a health crisis looming. The Chief Medical Officer, Donald Acheson, quickly realised the enormity of the problem and the possibility of it getting significantly worse. The prime minister at the time saw HIV as an economic risk and, realising the need for action, handed the problem to Norman Fowler, The Secretary of State for Health. Fowler coordinated a high-level political response through Cabinet committees and an emergency debate in the House of Commons in 1986, during which he emphasised the enormity of the crisis by announcing funding of £20 million for a public health campaign. Within the Tory government of the time, there was an absence of knowledge and no ready-made policies that could be adopted to address the increasingly feared epidemic. Seeing AIDS as a national public health emergency that needed to be handled especially sensitively led to an unprecedented meeting between Donald Acheson, Tony Whitehead from the Terrence Higgins Trust, Norman Fowler, and government ministers where lead clinicians and HIV charity workers were invited to inform the government of the current HIV position and its likely outcome.

To determine the extent of the HIV spread in the UK, an initial idea was to screen people, and to limit its transmission, add HIV to the list of notifiable diseases such as smallpox (Notification of Diseases Act, 1889) and isolate those infected. This gave rise to both fear and incredulity, as a gay activist, already knowing he was positive, joked:

> There was some … suggestion that we should all be isolated on an island, and I quite fancied somewhere like Barbados but that wasn't what they meant.

History had shown that in the attempts to control sexually transmitted infections such as syphilis and gonorrhoea, an approach using confidentiality rather than quarantine had worked best (Brandt, 1988). Attempts in the 1940s to understand the links between lung cancer and smoking (Doll and Hill, 1956) had introduced the concepts of relative risk and risk factors which had led to public health policies that focused on an individual's life-style and an individual's responsibility for their own health, rather than moral diktats, as described by a female policy maker:

> The parliamentary enquiry and the British Medical Association's evidence together were very influential in terms of setting the idea that… [the response] should be driven by a pragmatic, public health policy approach rather than by ideologies.

Acheson had the foresight to realise that to prevent the spread of HIV in gay men, the gay community had to be involved in prevention campaigns. Through patient advocates from the Terrence Higgins Trust, patients found their voices; an innovation reported by a policy maker:

> There was a shift in thinking … from 'we'll consult PLWH' to 'we'll involve them in the policy-making process from the outset'.

So, AIDS policy, response, and funding were developed using a scientific approach, through the powerful interaction of epidemiological (relative risk) and biomedical models of disease and were agreed by bureaucrats, rather than politicians, although, as a charity worker recalls, this wasn't always easy:

> There was real reluctance for the Civil Service to allow ministers to be seen to be being influenced by gay radicals … at that time if you were a lesbian or a gay man or volunteering for The London Lesbian and Gay Switchboard or THT, you were by definition a radical left winger.

Prevention

Discussions between the Chief Medical Officer and the Terrence Higgins Trust highlighted the need for preventative action and ring-fenced funding for those infected. Prevention through public health education was considered acceptable and economically sound by politicians as it would save on future care bills and was preferable to making free condoms widely available, a practice that could be viewed as promoting certain sexual behaviours.

After an initial newspaper advert in March 1986 giving advice, that was both obscure and had little impact (Fowler, 2014), a major sexual health campaign was proposed. This would be the first sexual health campaign since the Second World War. Although homosexual sexual acts in private had been decriminalised in the UK with the passing of the Sexual Offences Act in 1967, public attitudes towards homosexuality had not significantly shifted away from overwhelming homophobia, and as the epidemic was mainly in gay men, there was a desire to ensure the public were alerted without stoking prejudiced reactions. A policy maker described the difficulties they faced:

> There was a difficulty in saying 'well it's not a gay disease, anybody can get this' ... to actually acknowledging that it is the gay community that is most affected, and most needs our support ... and then the African communities who were largely asylum seekers and refugees. How we [could] handle the dynamic of acknowledging that certain communities are most affected whilst at the same time fighting against prejudice and stigma for those communities became a very difficult dynamic.

Initially, two campaigns were considered: one to address gay behaviours within the gay community, and the second to inform the general heterosexual population. Not everyone saw this as a non-prejudiced response, as the sceptical response of a gay activist demonstrates:

> They didn't want to get their hands dirty ... Surreptitiously, give some money to the poofters and allow them to get on with it.

Finally, only one general message went forward, detailing sexual behaviour rather than sexual orientation. This was accepted by the gay community as it justified their assertions that HIV was not a gay plague. However, the campaign was subsequently interpreted as the beginning of the de-gaying of AIDS (King, 1994). Within the recently formed Special AIDS Cabinet Committee there were divided views as to whether the message should focus on moral issues such as being faithful to one partner, or should come from a public health perspective, detailing risky behaviours and preventative measures. There was concern also over how explicit the messages should be. Again, information had to be clear enough to prevent infection whilst not stoking homophobia. There was no precedent for the appropriate way in which to describe the sexual acts involved in HIV transmission. Should one say, sexual intercourse, or having sex? Was it better to say anal sex, rectal sex, or back-passage sex? (Berridge, 1996). A gay activist recalls the discussions:

Nervousness if you used language … that could increase fear of people with HIV and [increase] stigmatisation … How do you inform without frightening in a way which has a backlash? We got a lot of information over from the States … Our key issue was, how do you get sex education out when you can't talk about sex? So that was one of our first fights.

Evidence from the First and Second World Wars showed that attempts to prevent the spread of syphilis and gonorrhoea in troops using messages that encouraged troops to resist temptation and to avoid intimacy, had not been successful, with 20% of those on leave in Paris during the First World War acquiring a sexually transmitted infection (Adler, 1980). In contrast, provision of practical advice and protection during the Second World War reduced infection in similar circumstances to 3% (Fowler, 2014). A campaign was planned in which a leaflet using explicit language that detailed the facts of HIV transmission would be delivered to every household, public posters would provide alerts, and TV and radio coverage would provide education. Organised by an advertising agency and civil servants without the input of any health education experts (Dorn, 1986) its success was not guaranteed. The 'Don't Die of Ignorance' leaflet – or as it is frequently referred to, 'The Tombstone' – reached 23 million households in March 1987 and was followed by a week of TV programmes – 'AIDS Week'. The campaign was directed at heterosexuals with no specific gay perspective. Whether or not this was the right decision was subsequently questioned. As a doctor reflected:

The tombstone adverts were part of that project fear … in making people aware … but that probably increased stigma. To a certain extent it was the right approach, but it also had its legacy.

Despite fears that TV and radio presenters might be limited by the government in what they could say, discussion of sexual practices and condoms in documentaries was accepted by the public and an empathetic response to those with HIV prevailed in the documentaries, although at the same time, there was a hardening in attitudes to homosexuals with criminalisation, sterilisation, and isolation being a few of the punitive responses advocated (*News of the World*, 1987). In the weeks following the TV campaign, large numbers of heterosexuals, having had sex without a condom, and not realising the difference between 'risk' and 'relative risk' (Porta, 2014) reported at sexual health clinics asking for an HIV test. With counselling and a negative HIV test result most were easily reassured but some remained unconvinced, despite repeated clinical and serological evidence to the contrary. These became known as the 'Worried Well'; as it transpired, somewhat inappropriately, as they frequently presented with a range of psychological difficulties (Miller, Acton, and Hedge, 1988).

Whether the campaign was effective is debatable. The extent to which a mass media campaign could bring about individual behaviour change was probably limited. It aimed to scare gay men into having safer sex. But, as both a charity worker and a gay man living with HIV recall, with first-hand knowledge that their friends were dying, there had already been a fundamental change in the sex lives of most gay men:

> *In many different ways; those who gave up sex completely, those who stopped having penetrative sex … and the uptake of condom use and its consistency … and that was community driven.*

> *There was a badge that you had to show[you] were a good gay as regards HIV, which was a pink triangle … taken from the concentration camp badges, but with two little safety pins through it, to [demonstrate] safe sex and how responsible you are being.*

For those experiencing difficulties in changing their sexual practices, making the necessary adjustments to their behaviours required more fundamental changes, such as increasing their assertiveness and negotiating skills, reducing sexual anxieties, and addressing perceived stigma. Counselling and clinical psychology services widened their remit to address factors associated with unsafe sexual practices, and information emphasising the acceptability and enjoyment of gay safer sex was provided by the voluntary sector. For example, THT produced and distributed 'Tales of Gay Sex' in 1991, illustrating safer sex in everyday situations as negotiated interactions between gay men. Rates of new gonorrhoea infections (symptoms of which occur a few days after infection) had revealed a significant decrease as early as 1983, just as the media reports of a gay-related illness had mushroomed, suggesting that many had promptly heeded safer sex messages (Weller, Hindley, Adler, and Meldrum, 1984).

There are two aspects to the prevention of transmission of HIV. First, assisting those who are already infected to not pass HIV to others, and second, helping those who are uninfected to remain uninfected. As well as the national prevention campaigns that targeted everyone, the sexual health clinics who typically had as their clientele those who were sexually active, took on a major role in prevention. Health Advisers, who traditionally had the role of contact tracing for sexually transmitted infections, saw their role evolve to that of counsellors. They were trained to give information and a supportive ear to those testing positive with the added agenda of preventing further transmission by clarifying information on HIV transmission and opening discussion of safer sexual practices with both those testing positive and those testing negative. Along with promotion of the use of condoms came suggestions for innovative ways of enhancing non-penetrative sex. Perhaps never had sex been talked about so explicitly in England!

There were concerns that adolescents with haemophilia not knowing their HIV status would be starting their sex lives without using protection and thus putting others at risk. The haemophilia services were not used to talking about sex, and this discussion was frequently shelved. However, at this time, with no effective HIV treatments, few children survived and for many years this issue generally remained unaddressed.

Concern was raised in 1986 that HIV would jump from drug users to the general heterosexual population. A community research project into drug-using behaviours had found that the sharing of needles and syringes was spreading HIV between drug users (Brettle et al., 1986). Before AIDS awareness it was common for needles and syringes to be shared, not only because pharmacists had been advised not to sell injecting equipment, but also because in Scotland it was not uncommon for the police to confiscate syringes supplied by the GP with the idea that such measures would reduce heroin use. The HIV prevention campaigns did not always influence drug users as intended; in the words of a former injecting drug user:

> *With all those adverts on the telly… very scary, so I just wanted to take more heroin to stop it.*

Providing sufficient needles and syringes to prevent sharing was an obvious solution (McClelland, 1986). This suggestion was not universally welcomed as the free distribution of injecting equipment directly contradicted the government's abstinence approach, and when presented to the Department of Health there was concern, and opposition from the Scottish Office, that the provision of clean needles and syringes would condone and encourage drug use. A doctor working with injecting drug users described a typical response he encountered from Scottish Ministers:

> *You shouldn't do it … it's wrong … We'll take the needles away and then they'll stop.*

However, with most drug users being sexually active and levels of condom use low, the fear was that their sexual partners could provide a bridge for HIV to pass into the wider heterosexual population. The impetus from physicians was for a 'harm reduction' approach, leading a policy maker to comment that the development of needle exchanges providing clean injecting apparatus became inevitable:

> *We knew this would be an intervention that would be technically effective, but we genuinely didn't know whether there would be adverse, unwanted consequences; what the impact on the extent of drug use would be.*

The harm minimisation approach was backed by the UK Advisory Council of Misuse of Drugs (Advisory Council on the Misuse of Drugs, 1988) who gave a strong recommendation that the threat of HIV to public and individual health was far greater than that of drug misuse. In the words of an academic:

> *[At the time] we were less concerned about the problems associated with their injecting drug use and much more concerned to prevent HIV… [I] really pushed the harm minimisation message.*

To prevent confrontation between those implementing the harm minimisation approach and those espousing the war on drugs ideology (that refused to concede any help to drug users), a policy maker described how the Special Cabinet AIDS

Committee (Stimson, Alldritt, Dolan, and Donoghoe, 1988) decided to proceed through funding pilot projects:

> *I asked the chairman of the Special Cabinet AIDS Committee and … his perfect political answer 'recommend we do pilot projects and they be rigorously evaluated'. Which is what we did.*

So, needle exchanges became established, eventually even in Scotland, aiming to minimise harm from drug injecting rather than attempting to cure drug users or eradicate drug use. By 1991 there were more than 200 operating in the UK that were well used by drug users and they distributed more than four million syringes a year (Stimson, 1991). This proved a massive achievement in difficult political circumstances and no doubt saved many lives.

Clinical care

By the mid-1980s the central London hospitals were seeing a constant flow of new admissions of people with HIV. The government, being concerned that HIV might be a world-changing infection, was determined to minimise the spread of HIV in the UK. After much reduced funding for the NHS in the 1980s, new ring-fenced funding was made available for the treatment of AIDS, and a senior doctor appreciated the opportunities this provided:

> *The managers and the government really pushed the boat out … were very helpful. Talked to us weekly about what we needed. HIV was the first disease where the more [patients] you saw, the more money you got. So, we found out what patients wanted, rather than what you thought they needed.*

With good financial incentives, hospital care changed, becoming more patient-centred – where both quality of life as well as length of life were recognised as important. Dedicated HIV wards and specialist clinics were opened, and new clinical posts were financially supported. Initially, these separate clinics were provided to protect patients from discrimination on open wards. A gay nurse emotionally recalled his experience:

> *The cubicle had a little square piece of glass … and other patients' relatives kept peering in, looking at the AIDS patient … I said, he's not an animal from a zoo.*

Funding also paid for certain routine investigations that general hospital services had initially been unwilling to provide, perhaps through fear of contamination of equipment or fear of contagion. But a senior doctor recalls attitudes changing once funding became available:

> *At the time nobody would bronchoscope [people with HIV] and so we did it ourselves … As money came for AIDS everybody started saying we'll help you with those and we'd say, well you didn't want to help us two years ago, we can do it ourselves, thank*

you very much.

Patients were generally positive about their experiences in the London specialist hospitals, although a gay activist understood that there was still little that could be achieved medically:

> *The medical care was as good as it could be at the time … It was just so inadequate; not because nobody worked hard, but because nobody knew what to do … You became sick, you had horrible diseases, and you died.*

In the 1980s most doctors were unused to dealing with young dying patients, especially *en masse*, and were ill-equipped to respond to the totality of their needs. With the lack of any cure they recognised the patients' needs for emotional and physical support and the importance of involving health professionals with additional skills. So began the development of multidisciplinary teams that included professionals such as clinical psychologists, psychiatrists, social workers, and dieticians. A gay activist commented on changes he saw:

> *Younger physicians were open to the idea that medicine isn't necessarily solely the domain of physicians … the attitude rapidly changed when the deaths were becoming overwhelming on the wards and the physicians didn't have much to offer … there was an [attitude] we need all the help, and a willingness to collaborate; that's when you got services coming into the wards and the community being allowed to provide services in the wards and work together and that was very good.*

While duration of life was limited by HIV, a doctor acknowledged that quality of life was made a priority through the support of the multidisciplinary team, customising support for each individual patient.

> *This [approach] was important … from diagnosis to death … everything the patient needed we would deal with.*

A gay activist highlighted the changes this brought about in doctor–patient relationships. Now, patients had a voice like never before:

> *HIV created a space in which a group of 'articulate' patients could come along and fill the space, and the medical professionals had to listen because they needed our knowledge of how to deal with it.*

With the knowledge that there was little that medicine could offer, a charity worker commented on how patients' engagements with their doctors varied, with some giving total responsibility to the medical teams, others actively seeking a cure:

> *Many just said, you're the doctor, just do [it], I'm not well. Others wanted to explore all of the alternative treatments that were available … with nothing else around, exploring ayurvedic medicine and whether a high dose of vitamin C was helpful [was something to be done].*

Living with HIV became a waiting game – anticipating the opportunistic infection from which they would not recover. With death as the inevitable outcome, many PLWH made radical changes to their lives. For some, the thought of a limited tomorrow gave them courage, not just working through a bucket list, but making major changes to their lives. With no need to worry about mortgages or pensions, people gave up safe jobs that they hated and took up new careers, doing what they had always wanted. Some found that volunteering to help others or participating in research studies provided a meaning to life and helped them to psychologically survive. Others reacted to HIV by giving up work and enjoying each day as if there were no tomorrow, spending at will knowing the credit card need never be paid off.

The multidisciplinary teams tried to maximise quality of life by facilitating easy access to effective interventions that complemented the medical treatments. Mental health support was primarily needed to help people live with their HIV, but as HIV could also affect the brain directly, through infections such as toxoplasmosis and tumours, complex cases of mental health issues such as manic episodes, and dementias in the final months of life were not uncommon. The fear that HIV would induce long-term dementias was widespread (Bredesen, Levy, and Rosenblum, 1988; Tannock and Collier, 1989).

Suicide statistics are unreliable, with coroners erring on the side of caution before citing suicide as the cause of death. However, there did appear to be an increased rate of suicides in those with HIV (Marzuk et al., 1988), and many who survived suicide attempts were referred for psychological or psychiatric support. Multidisciplinary team members were acutely aware of the possibility of suicide in those succumbing to yet another opportunistic infection, such as cytomegalovirus (CMV) eye disease that adversely affected their sight. A rapid response by the mental health services was vital.

Although psychological support was routinely provided within the multidisciplinary teams of most major HIV units, unfortunately, for those requiring help for major mental health issues, care was not always readily available. Initially there was resistance from psychiatric in-patient units to take individuals with HIV. It appeared that their staff were worried about infection. When additional monies were provided, and specialist support and education instigated, the general mental health services became more involved. A psychiatrist working in an HIV unit reflected on his experiences with transferring patients:

> The psychiatrists … didn't quite understand … if somebody that we'd been seeing had become very unwell, manic, or very depressed, or suicidal, it was a huge battle to get them admitted. Partly because they were terrified everybody was going to get infected. What happens? Do we tell the other members of staff? Do we tell the other patients? So, it was a huge problem getting people [appropriate support] in the early days.

For those in declining health, visits to the hospital were difficult and not always beneficial, as they and the doctors knew that nothing more could be done. If patients could be supported to live comfortably, rather than live in fear or with depression, then something had been accomplished. District nurses, community nurses, or as they became known, the Home Support teams, took medical and nursing care into homes. They set up parenteral nutrition, intravenous pain relief and supported partners and families with their grief and concerns. For many, the Home Support teams became their families: people who supported them whilst knowing all their problems, weaknesses, and difficulties, who could be trusted not to desert them and would frequently be with them at the end. But, taking HIV care outside the dedicated, discrete hospital wards into homes had the potential to advertise the presence of HIV. Many Home Support nurses ditched their uniforms and went in mufti in order to maintain the confidentiality of patients.

As well as the need for good medical and nursing support the need to make everyday reality more bearable was appreciated by those with HIV themselves and concerned others. This went beyond the remit of the NHS and here many charities and volunteers, including some families who had lost someone to HIV, stepped in to provide access to holiday homes, respite care, and complementary therapies. Whilst not curative, such approaches did ease the pain of everyday living, contribute to well-being, and highlight the importance of human touch. For many, the fear of contagion meant those around them, such as their families, rarely held or hugged them, and medical treatment, although hands on, was rarely pleasant. In the words of a nurse working in a hospice and of a gay activist receiving care:

> *We had complementary therapies ... aromatherapists, acupuncturists, herbal therapies ... the place always smelt so fabulous and it was part of people's care.*

> *Things that made you feel better like a nice massage ... However kind the medical staff are, what they do to you tends to be unpleasant; it's blood, blood transfusions, it's cutting you ... So, if someone has gentle healing hands and kindness ... that's rather nice.*

End of life care

As people approached the ends of their lives, they spent increasing time in hospital even when there was little that medicine could offer. In the 1980s most hospices were set up to provide for elderly terminal care, and some specifically funded to provide for those with cancer. Although some were supportive of the occasional gay man and his partner, there were no facilities for the multitudes of gay men dying with an infectious disease. As the numbers dying from HIV-related illnesses increased, some hospices quickly indicated that they would only accept people with cancer, not HIV. With the fear that there would be no suitable facilities for end of life care for those with HIV, a number of initiatives for dedicated HIV hospices were proposed, including that of transforming an old school building into the 24-bed London Lighthouse in North Kensington (Spence, 1996), and an independent Christian Hospital in Shoreditch, into the Mildmay Mission Hospital.

HIV hospices offered support to people in their dying days, but with the ups and downs in people's health it soon became apparent that dedicated support was required not only in the last weeks of a person's life but through the recurrent illnesses experienced following an AIDS diagnosis. So, as well as providing a safe place for those dying, hospices evolved to provide community, day, and respite care for those who were long-term ill. In London, the London Lighthouse and the Mildmay Mission Hospital became part of the standard care package for PLWH. They were praised by nurses working in both hospitals and hospices:

> *The London Lighthouse was very much at the forefront of defining what HIV terminal care was and we quickly realised ... it was also palliative care ... It was about maintaining quality of life for as long as possible.*

> *A lot of our patients were frequent flyers. There was funding for stays and people would come in for a week out of four ... That would give their partner or carer a break or [prevent] them from struggling at home on their own.*

With people's acute illnesses being dealt with in the hospitals, and recuperation being provided by hospices, for adequate long-term care to be maintained close links between hospices and hospital services were developed. This 'joined up' thinking and integrated care was achieved through two-way communication, not only through sharing information by letter and phone, but also by key personnel, both medical and psychosocial, extending their input over all sites. So began co-dependent services; neither could operate successfully without the other.

Stigma and discrimination

Over the years productive links became established between charities, the NHS, and social and faith workers. But not everyone was helpful. There was continued opposition to the rights of homosexuals and continued fear and prejudice towards those with HIV within certain sectors of the community. Despite the British Medical Association having established the principle that there was no right to refuse treatment to PLWH (DHSS, 1986), some GPs refused to have PLWH on their lists, and dental care was not always made available. Many religious organisations took a very negative stance on gay relationships and not all funeral directors would accept the body of a person who had died from AIDS, and some who did lacked sensitivity, as witnessed by a gay nurse:

> *There was someone handing out cards in the waiting room [of the HIV outpatient clinic] and it was the funeral directors from across the way.*

In 1988 the first edition of The National AIDS Manual (NAM), a directory of those who could be relied on for support, was published. It gave details of GPs and dentists who were accepting and non-judgemental to those with HIV, of Church officials who would conduct sympathetic funerals, of empathetic funeral directors and of those to be avoided. Unfortunately, the stigma attached to those with HIV frequently spread to those offering supportive services, as one gay cleric who conducted funerals for a number of people who had died from HIV found when he attended a Church meeting:

> *I was ostracised by many of my colleagues as 'Him who must have AIDS'. The media were fascinated by the HIV epidemic. They disseminated fear and panic though their sensational presentation of the ease of contagion while stirring up homophobia through horror stories of the 'gay plague'.*

The media happily published the uninformed thoughts of figures of the establishment. Needless to say, most of these were not complimentary, and in the words of a community nurse:

> *Wherever there was a story about HIV, it always had a negative slant to it. It was never anything other than scaremongering or implying fear.*

A widely reported and commented-on speech was that of the Chief Police Constable of Manchester, James Anderton, who described PLWH as 'swirling around in a cesspit of their own making' (*Guardian*, 1986). A rather famous person described the epidemic as twofold: those who deserved the illness as it was of their own making, and those 'innocent victims' who were not responsible and therefore both innocent and a victim whom we could feel sorry for. This played on the relief people found if they could separate themselves from the majority of those who became infected (gay men).

Being able to 'out' a celebrity as gay, or even better with HIV, would sell papers, not just the tabloids. When rumours spread that a celebrity might be being treated for HIV in a particular clinic or hospital, unscrupulous tactics were employed to confirm suspicions. Within clinics, confidentiality was paramount and two nurses recount how hard it was to maintain confidentiality:

> *The press was so invasive … they'd come in with a bunch of flowers and say, 'these flowers are for "Well-known person"' and you'd thank them, and they'd say, 'so you can confirm that person's here then?'*

> *In medicine people respect confidentiality but we went the extra mile to be extremely careful … with phone calls, with visitors. You had to be on your guard the whole time.*

Patients frequently used pseudonyms to prevent any paperwork inadvertently disclosing their HIV status. Some well-known people, who were patients at HIV clinics, were well aware of the possibility of being 'outed' and arrangements were made to admit them to the clinics through back doors, as it was known that the press was lurking outside. A gay professional described how he coped with clinic visits:

> *I was always aware if I was going to the clinic; I'd look round to see if there were any journalists lurking in cars outside, so I was always aware there was a potential danger.*

With all AIDS stories being of interest, news of any celebrity supporting PLWH publicly was widely published and did help to promote the information that HIV was not spread through social contact. The most widely reported and most influential promotion of this message was the visit of Princess Diana to open a dedicated AIDS ward in the Middlesex Hospital. Not only did she not wear gloves, but she touched sick people with AIDS while talking to them.

The public were keen to understand the unfolding HIV epidemic and specialised medical reporting was also given column inches and praised by a doctor, who acknowledged its great value:

> There were two medical correspondents who were responsible and infinitely sensible. They understood science … Most of the sensational reporting was not done by medical correspondents; it was around contagion, around gay men, about excluding gay men and herding them up.

The media did not give government an easy ride. TV documentaries were used by all to make their cases; doctors and scientists criticised the lack of government action and a number of articulate gay men were interviewed on television providing the public with positive images of openly gay people who previously had been invisible in society. A charity worker saw the opportunity this gave gay men:

> In 1986, 87, there were only four television channels, and so if we were on the 9 or 10 o'clock news you knew that most people in the country had seen it.

Activism

The negative and biased reporting of HIV almost certainly fuelled activism. The injustices and stigma towards PLWH energised some to fight for their rights. A hospice nurse saw the efforts that had been made by her patients:

> The gay men mobilised, became a force to be reckoned with. They went from being this ignored legislated-against group, to these fighting, loud people not being ignored.

The activism battle had many fronts: human rights, the right to equal care and access to drugs, the right to participate in drug trials and in the development of prevention programmes. Fighting for the human rights of PLWH required an openness of sexuality and HIV status rarely before seen. People attended Gay Pride knowing they would be 'outed'. Some PLWH left the hospital wards in wheelchairs to attend Gay Pride, which itself became an increasingly political event. A charity worker highlighted the importance of the label attached to a person who had been infected with HIV. Rather than being described negatively, people named themselves confidently:

> People with AIDS took a lot of encouragement from what pioneers in the United States had done … framing it as People living with AIDS, rather than AIDS victims.

A policy maker described how the fight against homophobia was also taken on by the establishment:

> We [The British Medical Foundation for AIDS] took the tabloid newspaper to the Press Complaints Commission because they'd published something saying it's only those nasty homosexuals; heterosexuals can't get HIV and they misrepresented evidence … They had to publish a retraction, in small print on the bottom of page 37 … but nonetheless it was a victory.

Being an activist was not easy for some who feared reprisals, but a gay man living with HIV describes how, as more people spoke out, it became easier for others to join the activist movement:

> I'd never been politically active before but [activism] became the new life that I was able to make for myself in which having HIV made sense.

Believing that there had to be effective treatment for HIV infection, the development and provision of effective medication became a key challenge for HIV activists. The activists went directly to drug companies demanding access to the latest treatments.

When it became clear that the infected blood products imported from abroad had included those collected from paid drug users and from gay benevolent donors in the US, anger towards the government for failing to ensure a safe blood supply (that had been promised since 1970), increased. The Haemophilia Society had been providing support and information groups since 1950. Now the Society mainly became concerned with seeking compensation for HIV infection more than with the provision of direct psychosocial support for those infected.

Prevention of further transmission of HIV was crucial but the government faced the difficult dynamic of acknowledging that certain communities were most affected and were wary of demonising those with HIV, particularly gay men, by messages that attributed blame or responsibility. However, the reality of HIV transmission could be best acknowledged by those with HIV. In the words of one gay activist:

> [Man's name] got it right. He said, us positive guys should be prevention activists because after all we're the ones who are spreading the disease. No one else could have said such a thing without being offensive.

At times, activists were criticised for being disruptive and taking their activities too far. Was it appropriate to throw condoms over the prison walls, or to smash the stands of drug companies promoting antiretrovirals at HIV-related conferences? A doctor reflected on how advances in HIV medications might have been slowed without such tactics:

> I think patient activism was on balance, a great good. But Act Up perhaps went over the top on many occasions, but I think most activism was extremely helpful.

What he had found impressive, was that great progress had been made for PLWH and for gay men through their own determination at a time when the country in general was not supportive:

> One of the great things with HIV is the way patient groups sorted themselves out, insisted on better food, insisted on liberal laws.

Although later some of the activities of activists would be seen as paternalistic as they battled for the rights of PLWH, rather than supporting people to fight for their own human rights, it seems that at the time this was a necessary first step in promoting advocacy.

A sober end to the decade

As the 1980s drew to a close the outlook was bleak. More than 13,000 people in the UK had been diagnosed with HIV and more than 2,000 had died. With no effective medications it was doubtful that the situation would improve. As many could remain symptom free for years after becoming infected, the effectiveness of prevention campaigns remained unknown. Despite an underlying pessimism, a positive focus on dignity and humanity prevailed with activists, HIV charities, and health professionals. Their efforts helped to make the lives of those living with HIV more tolerable, while keeping a relentless focus on the challenges presented by HIV.

References

Adler, MW (1980) The terrible peril: A historical perspective on the venereal diseases. *British Medical Journal*, 281(6234), 206.

Advisory Council on the Misuse of Drugs (1988) *AIDS and drug misuse, Part 1.* London, Her Majesty's Stationery Office.

Berridge, V (1996) *AIDS in the UK: The making of a policy, 1981–1994.* New York, Oxford University Press.

Brandt, AM (1988) AIDS in historical perspective: Four lessons from the history of sexually transmitted diseases. *American Journal of Public Health*, 78(4), 367–371.

Bredesen, DE, Levy, RM, and Rosenblum, ML (1988) The neurology of human immunodeficiency virus infection. *QJM: An International Journal of Medicine*, 68(3–4), 665–677.

Brettle, R, Davidson, J, Davidson, S, Gray, J, Inglis, J, Conn, J, … McClelland, D (1986) HTLV-III antibodies in an Edinburgh clinic. *Lancet*, 1(8489), 1099.

DHSS (1985) *AIDS—Information for doctors concerning the introduction of the HTLV III antibody test.* London, DHSS.

DHSS (1986) *AIDS, Booklet 3: Guidance for surgeons, anaesthetists, dentists and their teams in dealing with patients infected with HTLV III.* London, DHSS.

DHSS (1987) *On the state of the public health: The annual report of the chief medical officer of the department of health for the year 1986.* London, DHSS.

Doll, R, and Hill, AB (1956) Lung cancer and other causes of death in relation to smoking. *British Medical Journal*, 2(5001), 1071.

Dorn, N (1986) Media campaigns. *Druglink*, 1(2), 8.

Fowler, N (2014) *AIDS: Don't die of prejudice*. London, Biteback Publishing.

Guardian (1986) *The Guardian*, 18 December.

Hedge, B, Petrak, J, Sherr, L, Glover, L, and Slaughter, J (1992) *Psychological crises in HV infection*. VII International Conference on AIDS, Florence.

King, E (1994) *Safety in numbers: Safer sex and gay men*. London, Cassell.

Marzuk, PM, Tierney, H, Tardiff, K, Gross, EM, Morgan, EB, Hsu, M-A, and Mann, JJ (1988) Increased risk of suicide in persons with AIDS. *JAMA*, 259(9), 1333–1337.

McClelland, D (1986) *HIV infection in Scotland: Report of the Scottish Committee on HIV infection and intravenous drug misuse*. Edinburgh, Scottish Home and Health Department.

Miller, D, and Carne, C (1987) *Living with AIDS and HIV*. London, Palgrave Macmillan.

Miller, D, Acton, TM, and Hedge, B (1988) The worried well: Their identification and management. *Journal of the Royal College of Physicians of London*, 22(3), 158.

News of the World (1987) You say – Outlaw gays. *News of the World*.

Porta, M (2014) *A dictionary of epidemiology*. New York, Oxford University Press.

Public Health England (2018) *National HIV surveillance data tables*.

Richards, T (1986) Don't tell me on a Friday. *British Medical Journal (Clinical Research Ed.)*, 292(6525), 943.

Robertson, JR, Bucknall, A, Welsby, P, Roberts, J, Inglis, J, Peutherer, J, and Brettle, R (1986a) Epidemic of AIDS related virus (HTLV-III/LAV) infection among intravenous drug abusers. *British Medical Journal (Clinical Research Ed.)*, 292(6519), 527–529.

Robertson, JR, Bucknall, A, and Wiggins, P (1986b) Regional variations in HIV antibody seropositivity in British intravenous drug users. *Lancet*, 1(8495), 1435–1436.

Royal College of Obstetricians and Gynaecologists (1987) *Report of the RCOG sub-committee on problems associated with AIDS in relation to obstetrics and gynaecology*. London, Royal College of Obstetricians and Gynaecology.

Spence, C (1996) *On watch: Views from the lighthouse*. London, Cassell.

Stimson, GV (1991) Risk reduction by drug users with regard to HIV infection. *International Review of Psychiatry*, 3(3–4), 401–415.

Stimson, GV, Alldritt, L, Dolan, K, and Donoghoe, M (1988) Syringe exchange schemes for drug users in England and Scotland. *British Medical Journal (Clinical Research Ed.)*, 296(6638), 1717–1719.

Tannock, C, and Collier, C (1989) *We're just in time: AIDS, brain damage and psychiatric hospital closures: A policy rethink*. London, Bow Group.

The Times (1985) Boy in AIDS-risk case allowed into school. *The Times*.

Weller, I, Hindley, D, Adler, M, and Meldrum, J (1984) Gonorrhoea in homosexual men and media coverage of the acquired immune deficiency syndrome in London 1982–3. *British Medical Journal (Clinical Research Ed.)*, 289(6451), 1041.

3 Slow progress

Introduction

In 1988 the reality of a worldwide AIDS epidemic, including an acknowledgement of the scale of the problem in many African countries, led to the World Health Organisation (WHO) establishing the Global Programme on AIDS (GPA). The GPA provided a forum for disseminating worldwide AIDS prevention programmes, whilst promoting the US and UK traditions of liberal responses to those infected, including respect for individual rights, anti-discrimination policies and self-help. The *International AIDS Conference* became an established annual event, bringing together scientists, physicians, psychologists, psychiatrists, activists, and community, social and charity workers.

The following year the WHO estimated that there were 400,000 cases of AIDS across 145 countries with 100,000 of these in the US (World Health Organisation, 1989). In the UK, by the end of 1989 the number of AIDS cases reported had risen to 2,536, with about 80% having already died (Public Health England, 2018).

Through the 1990s the epidemic not only spread among gay men across the UK, but also among increasing numbers of heterosexual Black Africans, both men and women. Many had never been tested for HIV, and so their first hospitalisation was often with advanced disease, when there was little that medicine could offer.

The Department of Health now recognised that AIDS merited special attention and regular funding. Grants to health and local authorities rose from £25.1 million in 1987–1988 to £126 million in 1990–1991. More funding to statutory service providers, rather than to small and gay voluntary organisations, allowed an expansion of paid rather than volunteer posts. Many voluntary organisations then ran into financial and managerial trouble.

In addition to the research into vaccine development and therapeutic trials funded within the AIDS Directed Programme, in 1988 the AIDS Initiative contributed to AIDS policy development by promoting social epidemiological studies. The agreement to permit the anonymous screening for HIV in research studies in 1989 brought greater certainty to the estimates of HIV infection across the country and within different communities.

By 1988 better treatments for opportunistic infections were available, and in 1989 the concept of prevention of opportunistic infections by early treatment and primary prophylaxis was established. In particular, the licensing of aerosolised pentamidine for the prevention of Pneumocystis Carinii Pneumonia (PCP) was an important step. The first drug able to interfere with the replication of the virus directly, the antiretroviral azidothymidine (AZT), became available in 1987 and showed promise, as it initially improved the symptoms of many with advanced HIV disease (Barnes, 1986; Yarchoan et al., 1986). However, the Concorde trial, investigating the effectiveness of AZT in those with asymptomatic disease, which had started in 1988, brought disappointing results in the spring of 1993, when it was shown to have no effect on mortality or disease progression (Aboulker and Swart, 1993).

In 1989 the US initiated group ACT UP, the AIDS Coalition to Unleash Power, had its first meeting in London. It pushed for a much more rapid response to the development of treatments for those dying with AIDS, targeting drug companies, the government, and the press through public demonstrations and protests, with some success.

The legal case for compensation to people with haemophilia who had contracted HIV through contaminated supplies of factor VIII was settled out of court in 1990. Every person with haemophilia who was infected with HIV through the blood supply was awarded a payment of up to £60,000. The Haemophilia Society with the support of all political parties had successfully persisted in their claims for compensation driven by the injustice of deaths, as an activist with haemophilia reflected:

> *Only when John Major came in … it was his first act; he agreed an out of court settlement and they set up the Macfarlane Trust.*

As the haemophilia centres had switched to only using heat treated factor VIII (that destroyed HIV) in the autumn of 1985, new cases of HIV in people with haemophilia were consigned to the past.

In 1991, celebrities embraced and publicised their support for AIDS by adopting the Red Ribbon at US film and television award ceremonies. The Red Ribbon was launched in the UK at the tribute to Freddie Mercury who died with AIDS that year. Mainstream depictions of AIDS and gay men soon followed in 1993, with the major Hollywood film *Philadelphia* starring Tom Hanks, while Tony Kushner's play *Angels in America* won the Pulitzer Prize for drama.

After many years of presenting research findings on HIV and AIDS in sexual health forums, in 1995 the British HIV Association (BHIVA) was formed.

The epidemic spreads

As the numbers infected with HIV grew steadily through the late 1980s and early 1990s, so many more people presented to hospital with advanced disease, as a gay man living with HIV recalled:

> *Waking up that Saturday morning with a temperature through the roof … not just the sheets but the duvet being soaked through, the pillows being soaking wet … [The doctor said] you've got loads of fluid on the lung, you've got to come into hospital. They took me to the overflow HIV ward, that's how bad it was in 1994.*

Most of these people living with HIV (PLWH) lived in the London area or in Scotland. The minority who lived elsewhere in the UK tended to come to London for specialist treatment that guaranteed anonymity and confidentiality. But now, particularly where there was a significant gay population, such as in Manchester and Brighton, numbers testing positive grew, necessitating the establishment of local services.

A vast increase in government expenditure allowed services and posts to be developed in both the statutory and the voluntary sectors to meet the needs of all with, or affected by HIV, from diagnosis until death. Increases in the number of hospital carers, designated social workers, and home-care teams were apparent, with significant funding also reaching voluntary sector organisations. A person-centred service now became available to most PLWH. Monies for care were ring-fenced and allocated annually, based on the number of AIDS patients in each health- and local authority. Consequently, most funds went to the London health authorities, with all authorities receiving at least a small fund to estimate the current AIDS situation and its possible spread in their area. But as suspected at the time, and later documented (Comptroller and Auditor General, 1991), it does appear that while some Regional Health Authorities overspent their budgets, some diverted funds to other activities, such as offsetting capital deficits and funding hospital building programmes (Garfield and Davenport-Hines, 1995). Within the Expert Advisory Group on AIDS (EAGA), the Department of Health's initial and sole advisor, the balance of power altered: the AIDS experts, doctors, and scientists were no longer in the majority. An increase in the number of civil servants within the group allowed more government control over policy development (Karpf, 1988).

Integrated personal care

Many of those first infected with HIV had lived an urban and international travelling lifestyle, socialising with gay men across Europe and the US. Now HIV was spreading to wider gay circles globally, infecting those with a variety of lifestyles. HIV was not only prevalent in men who had sex with men, both those who identified as gay, and those who did not, drug users and men with haemophilia, but also in heterosexuals, particularly Black Africans, as became obvious to a gay man living with HIV:

> *And then for the first time, Africans with HIV that I was meeting.*

Evidence of the heterosexual spread of HIV accumulated. Sometimes, the whole family – man, woman, and children – would become ill. Their circumstances varied but a nurse described how it was not unusual to find people who had arrived in the UK whose HIV infection was only one amongst a host of problems they faced:

> *They were dealing with all sorts of things like torture from their previous countries and seeing a lot of people dying from HIV, very frightened, quite often isolated.*

Additional services and resources were needed to provide an appropriate response to the effects that trauma, escape, immigration, and asylum seeking superimposed on living with HIV. Support services that had been shaped to cater to the lifestyles of gay men now had to acquaint themselves with other kinds of difference, including the expression of non-Western cultures, heterosexual practices, and the meanings attached to parenthood (Nattabi, Li, Thompson, Orach, and Earnest, 2009). There was a particular need to distinguish mental health issues from a wide variety of health belief systems and ways of expressing emotions. A community nurse described how one immigrant responded to tooth ache:

> *He was labelled as a crazy person but a lot of this was cultural … He described the pain he was having as demons … but you realise his teeth are rotting out of his head … and he would say the demons are stabbing his mouth.*

By 1986 both wards and clinics offering specialised services for HIV had been set up with the needs of gay men paramount, while specific services for women had not yet been considered, as the experience of an activist with haemophilia showed:

> *When my girlfriend went for a [HIV] test in Swansea they said you can't come in here, this is the men's clinic … so we went to the women's clinic and they said, we don't do that test, so we had to go back to the men's clinic so she could have a blood test.*

Neither had the voluntary services or charities initially considered the needs of women with HIV as they had been instigated by gay men for gay men. With a small but significant increase in the number of women testing positive for HIV, charities were forced to reconsider their remit. A charity worker described how the Terrence Higgins Trust (THT) was challenged for being too 'gay' and not accepting of women:

> *Women finding the environment far too male, far too gay and not appreciating mothers … touched on deep things around sexism, misogyny, real or perceived, the sense that THT is not valuing women in the same way as it values gay men.*

Outside London there were no charity support services for women, and women experienced isolation. A community nurse reported that even in London, support for women was still limited, and women were at particular risk of isolation:

> *And the women had nobody. They were socially isolated. And dying in the same way.*

While in London, Manchester and Brighton those testing HIV positive were still predominately gay men, in Scotland the spread of infection was mainly through injecting drug use by both men and women, many of whom had children. A Scottish paediatrician described how from the beginning, their HIV services were set up to better provide for families, young people and children affected by HIV/AIDS:

> *There was the realisation that if you have drug users, a third of whom are women … these are women of child-bearing age … so by the time the clinic was set up in City Hospital, I was ready and we set up the first family clinic in the UK for children.*

The need for family care presented additional challenges. Like charities, many of the hospital wards had only seen gay men and were not equipped for women. Where single rooms were available, this was not a particular issue. But where PLWH were still accommodated on the old-fashioned Nightingale wards, complex decisions had to be made: when a mother was sick should she be separated from her child? How could children be accommodated in adult wards? Innovative solutions were called for and found. In London, for example, the Mildmay Mission Hospital opened a mother and baby unit providing tailored inpatient and day care. Because of ongoing drug use, ill health, or death, women could not always continue to care for their children. A paediatrician recalls how foster parents had to be found and vetted for children, some of whom had HIV:

> *I had to speak to prospective foster carers to de-stigmatise HIV, AIDS and how HIV is transmitted ... The foster carers were marvellous. They had no problems and welcomed the children into their homes.*

She described how children could face rejection even when they were not infected:

> *Schools were more problematic ... headline in the newspaper 'AIDS child goes to school' and the whole school would be cleared even though the child was not infected. I had to work with social workers, carers, teachers, and anyone who came into contact with children born to mothers with HIV.*

Even when AZT become available for adults, there was no specific drug regimen developed for children. With no alternative treatments available and despite the toxic effects well documented in adults, it was sometimes offered nevertheless. A paediatrician voiced her dilemma:

> *Sometimes you have no choice so you would have to explain to parents ... sometimes you would offer it and they would decline but where we did offer it, it was never effective.*

With the initial prediction that 50–75% of babies born to HIV-positive mothers would be infected (Minkoff, Nanda, Menez, and Fikrig, 1987; Scott et al., 1985), recommendations were that women with HIV should avoid pregnancy and that a termination would be available to those requesting it (Royal College of Obstetricians & Gynaecologists, 1987).

The desire for a child cannot be underestimated but the idea of bringing an infected child into the world was unthinkable to some. Both men who have sex with men (MSM), and heterosexual men and women with HIV reported strong desires for a child, and difficulty in coming to terms with self-enforced childlessness (Hedge and Sherr, 1989). However, not all women had the choice of preventing pregnancy, and those who for any reason found themselves already pregnant were offered the choice of a termination. Two women with HIV recounted:

> *But I'll never have children now, and that's terrible. I was 19.*

I had a few pregnancies; I had to get an abortion … My partner would insist on not using condoms.

For these continuing with a pregnancy the advice was to have a caesarean section, and follow up with AZT for the neonate, who should not be breastfed. A Black African woman described her experience:

She sent me off with all those pills … I eventually had the baby. They managed the labour covered in masks and what have you, so it was pretty weird … and then the child was on medication when born. [I was] not able to socialise … because you don't want to explain to anyone why you're not breastfeeding.

In some societies people are not viewed as adults until they had a child (Nattabi et al., 2009). With the push from the extended family for a couple to have a child, not having a child could 'out' them as possibly HIV infected; the factors influencing their behaviours were recognised by some, like this HIV policy maker:

[It was] difficult to get across the message that women don't necessarily have a choice about whether they use condoms or whether they have sex. The prevention messages focused on individual behaviour and not looking at the forces that shape behaviour.

Whether a child born to an HIV-positive mother was positive could not be known for some time, as initially babies carried the mother's antibodies. This was a trying time for doctors and parents who could do nothing other than watch and wait, as described by this paediatrician:

Follow-up was intensive – we were seeing babies at one week, three weeks and every six weeks until they were 18 months old when we could test them for HIV antibodies.

In Scotland two separate HIV services became established. One, based in the sexual health clinic was attended mainly by gay men, and the other was provided by select general practitioners (GPs), gradually evolved for drug users at Edinburgh's otherwise redundant City Hospital (following the decline of tuberculosis). With a core of staff already trained to manage infections and blood safely, this became the obvious place for an HIV testing site. Initially, drug users were reluctant to attend, fearing that they would be arrested. A doctor working with injecting drug users recalls how he gained their trust and attracted them, by assuring that those testing positive would have all their needs cared for:

People would come and see you because you're offering something they want and ultimately it moves on to providing drugs … But the start was we have to provide a service for people who have just been told that they're probably going to be dead in two years.

The development of medical services for drug users proved challenging. Their many needs were significant. Men, women, and children frequently existed in poor social and economic conditions. As drug users, there was a high probability that they would die from a drug-related incident, so little attention had been paid elsewhere to any additional problems that HIV presented. A 1987 paper (Des Jarlais et al., 1987), pointed to an association between higher frequencies of injecting behaviours and lower CD4 counts. This gave a rationale to restricting the supply of needles and syringes. Unfortunately, those who couldn't or wouldn't stop using drugs continued to share needles, getting them from wherever they could, as described by a doctor working with injecting drug users:

> *We had to keep our used needles and syringes in locked containers … people would steal stuff that had been used … out of the bins. You went, this is madness here.*

In some cities such as New York and Amsterdam, an alternative harm minimisation approach had been taken, with the provision of methadone to limit the need for injecting. Eventually, the UK medical services took on methadone prescribing. However, this moved the financial burden from the GP to the hospital. In an attempt to reduce the hospital budget, a doctor raised concerns when it was then proposed, that methadone should only be prescribed for those already HIV positive:

> *I said, but you realise you're telling people to go out and catch HIV? … If you're positive I'll give you methadone; if you're eligible come and see me; if you're not positive, clear off.*

With the media reporting the failings of this policy, the provision of maintenance methadone for all drug users became part of the public health model of harm reduction. The HIV screening services eventually morphed into services that met the medical and personal needs of drug users with HIV. As drug users are not always able to be organised, rather than expecting patients to fit in with the service, a psychiatric nurse described how services were developed around their users:

> *Giving a drug user an appointment at 9 am and expecting them to turn up is ridiculous. [The consultant] had the vision to set up a clinic that ran all day … Instead of expecting the patients to fit in with us, we developed a service around them. They would pitch up at some point convenient to them and they would be seen … In addition, other consultants like gynaecology, neurology, dermatology, ophthalmology would be on site. So, it was a kind of one-stop shop.*

Over time the unmet mental health needs of drug users with HIV became increasingly apparent. The local psychiatric services did not see caring for those with drug addiction within their remit, so dedicated psychiatric and psychological services were incorporated into the one-stop shop. A nurse highlighted the invaluable role played by local volunteers:

> *Charity [volunteers] existed to provide practical help. They would bring patients to their appointments. They would take them shopping. They would babysit for their children … all sorts of things that made a big difference to their lives. If necessary, they'd go via the chemist to pick up their methadone.*

The provision of a continuity of good, personalised care from doctors and nurses was reportedly a new experience for many of the drug users at the time. They had often come from abusive backgrounds and were not accepted by society at large. In the words of a doctor working with infected drug users:

> *They weren't used to people being friends with them. Sitting and chatting and asking them what was going on.*

Vaccines and treatments

To curtail the widespread transmission of HIV, the development of an HIV vaccine became one of the first priorities of the AIDS Directed Programme in 1987. It provided the Medical Research Council with monies for the basic science needed to develop an AIDS vaccine, with a view to a vaccine being developed within five years. This proved to be an insurmountable challenge, and with no significant progress, treatments for the opportunistic infections to which people became increasingly susceptible as their immune systems became impaired, became increasingly important.

Primary prophylactic treatment against many opportunistic infections such as PCP, became standard for those with low CD4 counts (Centers for Disease Control, 1989). This undoubtedly helped, but this treatment did not directly attack the virus. The first drug to be used against the virus directly, an antiretroviral, AZT, had been developed in the US and was approved for use in UK in 1987. There was initial optimism as it improved people's health at the outset, and so patients were willing to live with the side-effects and to adhere to the taxing four hourly regimen, even waking in the night and setting alarms to ensure they took every dose at the prescribed time. Doses given were high, and were not adjusted to the gender or weight of the patient, resulting in some smaller men and women experiencing particularly severe side-effects, including anaemia that required regular blood transfusions. However, as a female patient described, some took matters into their own hands, adjusting their medication regime:

> *He gives me AZT and tells me to take six … I took two … I thought there's no way I can take the same drug as a 12-stone man.*

Before long, the limited effectiveness of AZT and its severe side-effects became apparent, and a campaign against the use of AZT ensued. A gay nurse recalled the anger:

> *Some of the activists were angry with the doctors and pharma, we want AZT, then later, you're poisoning us with AZT.*

Despite a growing awareness of the limitations of AZT, HIV physicians continued to prescribe it. There was the hope that by keeping a person alive for longer, they had the chance to benefit from future medications. A doctor talked of the dilemmas they faced:

We thought we were doing the right thing, but we were also the enemy because we weren't doing it fast enough. We were using drugs that kill people. AZT equals death. But at the same time people with placards [demanded], why hasn't the FDA [Food and Drug Administration] approved AZT for more patients?

Although the development of successful antiretrovirals seemed slow to those who needed it, by 1991 other antiretroviral drugs such as ddC and ddI had become available. Once again, despite initial optimism, similar patterns of response emerged; initially drugs showed some benefit, but these benefits then faded. What became clear was that over time the virus was mutating and becoming resistant to each drug in turn, thus failing to improve a person's health. The limitations of treatment were summed up by a gay activist, already infected with HIV, and a hospice nurse:

Each time there was a treatment it really wasn't very good … so, basically the only options you had were fairly toxic drugs that gave short-term benefits … that was all they could do.

They were horrible drugs … people became resistant to the drugs or they died. Now, some good times but still waiting to die … but that was all there was, and it helped.

By 1990, routine CD4 counts were readily available to give a picture of the strength of a person's immune system and the trend of the disease. Whilst valuable in indicating when an immune system was so impaired it was unlikely to defend successfully against life-threatening infections, the CD4 count did not relate specifically to viral activity (amount of HIV circulating in the body) and proved a less than reliable surrogate marker of the effectiveness of an antiretroviral. The addition of routine viral load measurements in the early 1990s gave a much better indication of when an antiretroviral was proving successful and when it was failing. To maintain an 'undetectable viral load' was the aim of every PLWH.

At this time there was much concern that HIV would attack the brain. An American study in 1986 (Navia, Jordan, and Price, 1986) had estimated that 30–40% of those with an AIDS diagnosis would progress to dementia. It was suggested that reopening some of the recently closed psychiatric hospitals would provide suitable mental health beds for those with AIDS (Tannock and Collier, 1989). It is doubtful that the requirements of those with both the complications of advanced HIV disease and brain impairment could ever have been met by the old rundown Victorian psychiatric hospitals (Catalan and Riccio, 1990). Although neurological symptoms were apparent in many towards the end of their lives, the feared rise in cases of AIDS Dementia Complex failed to materialise, as a psychiatrist explained:

What happened was that those who first described the AIDS dementia complex had a very low threshold for impairment, so if you had a bit of confusion, if you couldn't walk properly, and were a bit aggressive, they would say it's [AIDS] dementia complex. They over diagnosed.

Drug trials

As discovery of an effective treatment against HIV was vital, a plethora of drug trials were set up to see whether the poor clinical outcome of untreated HIV infection could be changed. Initial studies had shown that a number of possible drugs were too toxic to be tolerated and that some combinations of drugs led to major negative drug interactions. But as PLWH realised they were going to die anyway, they pressed for access to the potentially useful new drugs, realising that they had little to lose even if they proved unsuccessful. This brought about a demand for adaptations to be made to the traditional approach of random controlled trials, in which a potentially active drug would be tested against a placebo. A gay nurse reflected that with the likelihood of death looming, many PLWH weighed up the possible benefits of a new trial drug against the risks to their own lives of taking potentially dangerous medications:

> *This guy goes, 'I know this [trial drug] may kill me but it will help the next lot; I'm going to die anyway.' These guys were brave.*

At the same time there were stories emerging from the US that people were both falsifying their medical records in order to gain entry to drug trials, and testing their allotted drugs, and subsequently leaving the trials if they had received placebos (France, 2016: 371). Thus, to find better ways to conduct drug trials became imperative. With the willingness of PLWH to participate in drug trials, charities and activists made clinical trial design a focus of their attention and sought representation on panels developing trials to ensure the needs of their communities could be met. A senior charity worker recalled:

> *So, Body Positive, The Haemophilia Society, THT [protested outside the BMA] demanding faster, bigger trials, more investment, a say in how the investment was used, what were the priorities and how the trials should be delivered.*

After many battles between AIDS activists, the FDA, and drug companies in the US, PLWH and their spokespeople became better represented on committees planning the design and development of clinical drug trials. Patient-centred changes to trial design were made, such as modifications to allow those on placebo to move to the active drug if their disease advanced, or trials only to compare different strengths of a new drug, e.g. the Alpha trial of ddI only compared the effects of high and low doses. This unprecedented, fundamental shift in the design of clinical trials benefited both research and patients, although it brought criticism from many scientists who thought such trial results of little use, and brought about conflicts between those who valued the traditional scientific method and those who put the humanity of individual patients first. But, by involving PLWH in the design and development of trials, many more PLWH volunteered and endeavoured to keep to trial protocols (France, 2016).

Living with HIV

As opportunistic infections were vigorously treated and increasingly prevented with prophylactic medications, those infected with HIV faced uncertain times. Whilst well, PLWH could find it difficult to imagine that these might be the last days of their lives, but as friends and acquaintances continued to die, there was ample evidence that once a diagnosis of AIDS had been given, few people lived more than a few years, as illustrated by the experience of a gay man living with HIV:

> *Turning up at the AIDS ward and seeing somebody you last saw on a dancefloor at a nightclub or at a sex party a year previously and dying in a wheelchair and I just wanted to stay away from it all.*

How people adjusted to the knowledge that they were infected with HIV varied. Some avoided addressing the issue, avoided medical check-ups and the few available treatments; others decided the future was too bleak to contemplate and took their own lives. Many, with the support of counsellors, mental health professionals, and voluntary groups redefined their lives and found meaning and enjoyment in their final years. A gay man living with HIV described the change he made:

> *You try to shift your life from this long-term perspective of what you're going to do and eventually you'll get old and you'll retire ... but you focused on short-term things to make life as good as possible.*

But life would never be the same again for those infected. For instance, with the knowledge that one could transmit a fatal disease to another through sex, there were far-reaching implications for PLWH in how they conducted their relationships and sex lives. A gay man talked about the logistics of managing sex:

> *I was someone who enjoyed going to clubs and pubs and that whole kind of lifestyle ... and I had absolutely no idea how to set about incorporating this news [being HIV positive] about myself; I had to be responsible. And the kind of sex I was having ... it wasn't something you went home and you had a cuppa and you discussed; the thought of telling somebody that you wanted to wear a condom because you [had HIV], it was just impossible.*

Levels of distress in those infected with HIV but still asymptomatic were high, with people experiencing anxiety, depression, relationship problems, adjustment to their HIV status, multiple bereavements, employment difficulties, sexual concerns, isolation, and suicide thoughts and ideation (Hedge and Sherr, 1995). But the greatest fears concerned death, as highlighted by this nurse:

> *Patients worried about how they were going to die. They certainly worried about getting dementia. They worried about going blind. Well they worried about dying. Who doesn't?*

Coping well with HIV infection seemed to be associated with continued good physical health and adoption of a proactive style including problem solving, expression of feelings, seeking emotional support, and taking control wherever possible, rather than falling into helplessness and denying fears (Hedge, Slaughter, Flynn, and Green, 1993; Remien, Rabkin, Williams, and Katoff, 1992). In the words of an activist with haemophilia:

> *It only took a few years for me to realise that with AIDS what happened was once you got ill three years later you died … so, if I was healthy, I should do stuff.*

Once HIV-related symptoms appeared, it became more difficult for people to remain hopeful (Kessler et al., 1988). Becoming ill had many ramifications, both practical and psychological, as these experiences of gay men with HIV showed:

> *I began to feel quite ill, quite stressed, and then … I had a lump beginning in my belly and I thought oh it's a cyst, it's nothing … but I was getting tireder and tireder … so I decided to come back to England … and that was the start of a whole new chapter for me, because I was suddenly homeless, penniless, without a lover, and on an AIDS ward.*

> *It was just after Christmas … and that's when it dawned on me. The money was running out and we were living in a sublet council flat. And the council was doing tenancy checks and so the housing had become very unstable. This is early 1992 and the precariousness of my situation started to dawn. The pain really started to intrude – emotional pain.*

Whether or not to take the available antiretrovirals was not an easy decision. With rumours about horrific, multiple side-effects associated with the new antiretrovirals some, like this man with haemophilia, decided not to take them, while others, like this heterosexual man saw the drugs as his only hope for survival:

> *I was very resistant to taking any treatment. My argument was that it would ruin the quality of my remaining life without extending it significantly. It's not going to cure the problem; it's just going to prolong an unpleasant [experience].*

> *My liver was enlarged, and they took me off AZT … Although some people done OK and all this question over AZT, I'd do the same thing again, I grabbed it with both hands. There was nothing else. I was on my last legs. I had a CD4 count of two.*

Not surprisingly, a wide range of mental health problems have been documented in PLWH, across all stages of infection, from diagnosis until death (Hedge and Sherr, 1995; Ostrow et al., 1989). In the words of a young gay man:

> *We were all in our late 20s and it was the first time of having to deal with the potential illness and mortality in your age group, big heady things … and we just weren't emotionally prepared to deal with it and although I was in a very safe space I was feeling really quite isolated and I become very lonely … and I started to become very depressed, not a bit blue … it was proper clinical depression. I was depressed for two years before I got any help.*

Funding for psychological support had been made available to the multidisciplinary hospital HIV teams and to many voluntary organisations. It became clear that some PLWH required immediate support as they faced a crisis, and the majority benefited from an individual, focused therapy lasting three to six months. At the same time the provision of support groups flourished, many provided by the voluntary sector. These frequently complemented individual therapeutic support (Hedge and Glover, 1990). However, not having disclosed an HIV infection to anyone outside the health care system meant that many found the prospect of going to an HIV-specific support group daunting. A gay man described his experience:

> *I remember going to the door feeling absolutely petrified … it would be the first time that I'd gone anywhere … where there would be an HIV label on you, and you would be saying 'I have HIV' by going into this room. It was very frightening … it's possible that there might have been somebody else who knew me, and the news would be out of my control potentially over who could find out.*

However, the experience of meeting others with HIV frequently proved not only therapeutic but also gave group members a sense of control over their lives. Rather than remaining alone with their fears, allowing an illusion that they were the only one infected, accessing a support group helped people connect to others with similar concerns and predicaments. Group attendance was praised by both a man with haemophilia and a gay man:

> *I went to the local Body Positive group; it was the best group I've ever been involved in, the most supportive, the most fun, the most enjoyable. [It included] three gay men, one ex-heroin user, and a single mother so we met at her house, so she didn't need child-care.*

> *The most important thing was just knowing that you weren't on your own with it [HIV] and that there were other people like you who went out to clubs and who were going through exactly the same experience not knowing how you were going to cope and thinking is there any kind of life for me after this. Simply hearing that other people were going through the same thing was probably at that point life changing, in that for the first time I thought, oh well, if other people are having to do this maybe I can do it and maybe we can help each other.*

Fears and discrimination

Although the transmission routes for HIV were now well established, there were still instances of irrational fear, even within the healthcare system. This seemed to be most prevalent when the fate of an unborn child was in question. Whether pregnant nurses should care for PLWH was questioned. Were they seen as more vulnerable, less likely to adhere to universal precautions or just important because of the foetus? A community nurse described concerns when she was pregnant:

> *The consultant said, well I don't think you should be working in this field [nursing] while you're pregnant … Some nurses [asked] do you have to wear a mask when you're seeing patients while you're pregnant?*

Some healthcare workers did have difficulty in accepting the lifestyle and sexual practices of gay men, but many more were judgemental about drug users. Ignoring the factors that may have contributed to the use of drugs, many users were seen to have brought HIV on themselves. A nurse and a doctor working with injecting drug users commented that drug users could be hard to empathise with, as their behaviours, such as unsafe sex with partners and with those they met while travelling (e.g. to Thailand, in order to score drugs), were not always easy to respect:

> *I think we were good at treating gay men but … sometimes a bit judgemental about drug users … sometimes they were a challenge. If they are currently using … issues about dealing in the day room and issues about abusiveness.*

> *[Drug users] weren't that nice … they were violent, self-centred people … it was difficult for them to learn to behave acceptably to the staff.*

Compensation for people with haemophilia who had been infected with HIV had been achieved by the Haemophilia Society with the support of THT, as per an agreement reported by a gay charity worker below. And despite the hardships suffered by gay men living with HIV, an activist with haemophilia reported that there did not appear to be any bitterness attached to these payments:

> *We did a deal; if the Haemophilia Society never uses the innocent victim tag, never claims that we are the innocent victims of AIDS, we attempt to give structured support to their case for compensation [for] having been infected through the health service. I can't ever remember any gay man saying it's not fair that you get money and I don't … I actually felt guilty about it.*

But a gay charity worker suggested that not all kept to the agreement to not discriminate against other groups of PLWH:

> *The Haemophilia Society stuck to that. Individuals with haemophilia didn't … there's always good AIDS, bad AIDS and very, very bad AIDS.*

Progress

But progress was being made. Funding had been made available for treatment and care. The government had provided a lead, protecting PLWH from victimisation and punitive measures. Despite all of the horrors of the epidemic, a patient-centred, multidisciplinary healthcare system for PLWH had developed, integrating NHS medical, psychological, social, and psychiatric care, with charity support, together with people's drug and spiritual needs. The huge emotional impact on those infected had resulted in an emotionally challenging but supportive environment that met patients' needs. A female academic described how this was generally welcomed:

> *There was always a multidisciplinary approach … though it was contained in the hands of a few small tight-knit groups which had the benefits of great care and a lot of innovation … but maybe closed to some ideas.*

Uniquely, PLWH had been involved in the planning and delivery of their own care. This is common practice now for people with many conditions such as cancer and diabetes, but as a doctor recognised, HIV services were at the forefront of this kind of patient-centred care:

> *One of the major positives about HIV care has been patient engagement through peer support services.*

There were by now two reliable markers that enabled a person's HIV health to be assessed accurately. These were also to become useful in drug trials, quantifying the response to potential new antiretrovirals. In the words of a doctor:

> *With HIV we were very lucky that, about the time the drugs became effective, it became clear that the two surrogate markers, the CD4 count and the viral load, were very accurate to predict the outcome.*

There was a huge engagement from those infected with HIV willing to take part in drug trials. The altruism of those knowing they were becoming sicker and would die volunteering for drug trials was an inspiration.

The general horror of HIV led to services being seen as apart from the mainstream hospital services. As a consequence, those working in the field often saw themselves as different, as belonging to an AIDS community. With high levels of bonding and support within teams (as opposed to the traditional hierarchical medical structure), and between staff and patients, the traditional distance between patient and doctor fell away. Christmas celebrations were no longer 'staff parties' but ward parties where staff and patients celebrated together, and charities brought in entertainment that might have been considered risqué elsewhere. But the unrelenting numbers of new infections, of those becoming sick and dying with HIV took its toll on professionals and volunteers. A gay activist recalled how this particularly affected those like himself infected with HIV:

> *It was incredibly stressful but it was an issue of survival so you weren't able to sit back and think [not help this week] because next week it might be you in that bed. So it was all hands on deck, and it was intensely stressful and traumatising.*

While HIV services had grown, and celebrities had endorsed HIV charities, not all health services had prospered. Some resentment was shown towards AIDS services, maybe exacerbated by their self-contained nature. A charity worker observed:

> *There was a kickback amongst arguably AIDS-phobic and homophobic medical establishment and research staff who would say, 'Why is all this money going to AIDS? AIDS gets all the money; AIDS gets all the attention'; that was difficult to manage.*

But as a senior doctor recognised, services had not been developed through messages of helplessness; rather, dedicated and talented individuals had donated years of hard work to the problem:

Why is HIV getting all the money? … In part that was because of the speed with which we'd shown we could describe, analyse, embrace and then start solving the problems.

But some difficult relationships between medical departments did ensue once money was available. For example, there were disputes over the funding of social work, psychological, and psychiatric support for children with HIV. The paediatricians claimed their funding was for oncology and that paediatric support for children with HIV should come from HIV funds, and not drain their resources. In the words of a paediatrician:

I said it will be really nice if some of the social work services, and the psychological and psychiatric support could be offered to the children with HIV. I was told you're lucky because there's all this funding available for HIV and that's where you should be going, not drain on our services.

The initial mass media prevention campaigns organised by Norman Fowler in 1986 and 1987 had emphasised risky sexual behaviours, and not focused on the most affected groups such as gay men. At the time this approach had the advantage of reducing the public view of the 'gay plague' and subsequently HIV funding had been allocated across all sectors of society. Prevention campaigns continued to focus on changing the sexual and drug-using behaviours of individuals with little attention to underlying social factors. By 1989 it became clear that although the number of infected heterosexuals was rising, the main UK epidemic remained in gay men. However, no specific funding or prevention campaigns targeted gay men. The initial funding provided through the AIDS Division of the Health Education Authority (HEA) took approximately 40% of the HEA budget and with the claims for support for other diseases, this could not be sustained. Changes were made to the organisation of funding within the HEA so that funding for HIV was incorporated into its sexual health programme. This led to the end of ring-fenced funding for HIV, and within the sexual health programme funding easily became diffused.

Where will it end?

1995 could be viewed as the nadir of HIV with the fears of a worldwide, unstoppable pandemic being realised. The trickle of patients seen in 1981 by the London hospitals had been steeply increasing since 1986. By 1995 nearly 3,000 people, 80% of them gay men, had been diagnosed with HIV in the UK (Public Health England, 2018). The enormity of the problem was described by a hospital doctor:

Suddenly, [numbers] exploded … you could estimate that you had 10% of your patients in hospital at any one time. If we extrapolate that to now, we would have 12,000 people in hospital with AIDS at any one time.

As the number of people infected, and the numbers dying with no effective treatment, continued to rise, there came the requirement for more inpatient facilities, more dedicated HIV wards, and more hospice care.

Counselling, psychological and psychiatric services were inundated with those realistically seeing their lives drawing to a close and striving to maintain some quality to their last days. The fear of a scenario of huge numbers of people living with AIDS-related brain diseases remained, despite evidence showing that most people with severe brain impairment died before long-term care was required.

Over the years there had been a proliferation of charities in an increasing number of cities throughout the UK, each believing they could support people in a unique way or cater to a specific community. Many expanded rapidly but with a lack of managerial experience, and with attempts to add new services to their original remit of providing individual voluntary support, not all prospered. Competition between them for resources became evident and a charity worker recognised the difficulties ahead:

> *All fighting for funding … Lack of clarity as [to] what differences between groups were. How they could remain active was not always clear.*

There were a number of attempts to coordinate the efforts of the voluntary sector organisations but with continuing power struggles between providers and no national lead, the mainstream funding made available for professional psychological and social support increased and less became available for the HIV-related charities.

As HIV became mainstream, charities may have had less access to government funding and less influence on HIV-related policies but HIV started to attract support and funds from society celebrities and businesses who were pleased to add their names to the HIV cause, supporting new initiatives such as the London Lighthouse, a dedicated HIV hospice.

As well-known personalities became willing to support HIV-related causes, more in the population not directly affected by HIV were willing to openly show their support and the World AIDS Day became an annual event with symbolic red ribbons becoming the international symbol of support for the HIV cause, being distributed widely throughout the country. Although clinical trials for new antiretrovirals continued there were frequent disappointments. People were living longer, but they were still dying after experiencing disabling physical and major mental illnesses. However, one charity worker did see a glimmer of hope:

> *The Concorde trial results were depressing … The number of people being diagnosed continued to rise. The number of funerals continued to grow … but already, even then, the first seeds … that dual combination therapy being more effective than AZT on its own was known.*

References

Aboulker, J-P, and Swart, A (1993) Preliminary analysis of the Concorde trial. *The Lancet*, 341(8849), 889–890. doi:10.1177%2F1440783309335650

Barnes, DM (1986) Promising results halt trial of anti-AIDS drug. *Science*, 234, 15–17.

Catalan, J, and Riccio, M (1990) We're just in time–AIDS, brain damage and psychiatric hospital closures: A policy rethink. *Psychiatric Bulletin*, 14(11), 694–696.

Centers for Disease Control (1989) Guidelines for prophylaxis against Pneumocystis carinii pneumonia for persons infected with human immunodeficiency virus. *MMWR Supplements*, 38(5), 1.

Comptroller and Auditor General (1991) *HIV and AIDS related health services*. London, Her Majesty's Stationery Office.

Des Jarlais, D, Friedman, SR, Marmor, M, Cohen, H, Mildvan, D, Yancovitz, S, … Garber, J (1987) Development of AIDS, HIV seroconversion, and potential co-factors for T4 cell loss in a cohort of intravenous drug users. *AIDS (London, England)*, 1(2), 105–111.

France, D (2016) *How to survive a plague: The story of how activists and scientists tamed AIDS*. London, Pan Macmillan.

Garfield, S, and Davenport-Hines, R (1995) The end of innocence: Britain in the time of AIDS. *Nature*, 373(6509), 29–29.

Hedge, B, and Glover, L (1990) Group intervention with HIV seropositive patients and their partners. *AIDS Care*, 2(2), 147–154.

Hedge, B, and Sherr, L (1989) *On becoming a mother: Counselling implications for mothers and fathers. International conference on the implications of AIDS for mothers and children*, WHO, Paris.

Hedge, B, and Sherr, L (1995) Psychological needs and HIV/AIDS. *Clinical Psychology & Psychotherapy*, 2(4), 203–209.

Hedge, B, Slaughter, J, Flynn, R, and Green, J (1993) *Coping with HIV disease: Successful attributes and strategies. IX International AIDS Conference*, Berlin.

Karpf, A (1988) *Doctoring the media: The reporting of health and medicine*. London, Taylor & Francis.

Kessler, RC, O'Brien, K, Joseph, JG, Ostrow, DG, Phair, JP, Chmiel, JS, … Emmons, C-A (1988) Effects of HIV infection, perceived health and clinical status on a cohort at risk for AIDS. *Social Science & Medicine*, 27(6), 569–578.

Minkoff, H, Nanda, D, Menez, R, and Fikrig, S (1987) Pregnancies resulting in infants with acquired immunodeficiency syndrome or AIDS-related complex: Follow-up of mothers, children, and subsequently born siblings. *Obstetrics and Gynecology*, 69(3 Pt 1), 288–291.

Nattabi, B, Li, J, Thompson, SC, Orach, CG, and Earnest, J (2009) A systematic review of factors influencing fertility desires and intentions among people living with HIV/AIDS: Implications for policy and service delivery. *AIDS and Behavior*, 13(5), 949–968.

Navia, BA, Jordan, BD, and Price, RW (1986) The AIDS dementia complex: I. Clinical features. *Annals of Neurology: Official Journal of the American Neurological Association and the Child Neurology Society*, 19(6), 517–524.

Ostrow, DG, Joseph, JG, Kessler, R, Soucy, J, Tal, M, Eller, M, … Phair, JP (1989) Disclosure of HIV antibody status: Behavioral and mental health correlates. *AIDS Education and Prevention*, 1, 1–11.

Public Health England (2018) *National HIV surveillance data tables*.

Remien, RH, Rabkin, JG, Williams, JB, and Katoff, L (1992) Coping strategies and health beliefs of AIDS long term survivors. *Psychology and Health*, 6(4), 335–345.

Royal College of Obstetricians & Gynaecologists (1987) *Report of the RCOG sub-committee on problems associated with AIDS in relation to obstetrics and gynaecology*. London, Royal College of Obstetricians and Gynaecologists.

Scott, GB, Fischl, MA, Klimas, N, Fletcher, MA, Dickinson, GM, Levine, RS, and Parks, WP (1985) Mothers of infants with the acquired immunodeficiency syndrome: evidence for both symptomatic and asymptomatic carriers. *Jama*, 253(3), 363–366.

Tannock, C, and Collier, C (1989) *We're just in time: AIDS, brain damage and psychiatric hospital closures: A policy rethink*. London, Bow Group.

World Health Organisation (1989) *HIV seropositivity and AIDS prevention and control*. Geneva, WHO.

Yarchoan, R, Weinhold, K, Lyerly, HK, Gelmann, E, Blum, R, Shearer, G, … Klecker, R (1986) Administration of 3'-azido-3'-deoxythymidine, an inhibitor of HTLV-III/LAV replication, to patients with AIDS or AIDS-related complex. *The Lancet*, 327(8481), 575–580.

4   Hope rising and the fallout

Introduction

The year is 1996, and momentous changes are about to take place, as described by a clinical psychologist, who witnessed first hand the announcement of new and encouraging research results:

> I actually went to the 1996 Vancouver International AIDS Conference and I was at the talk where they announced the results of the trials, and I can remember just being overwhelmed … it was amazing but it was also quite sad because there were some people who had, I knew, died that summer, and you think, for God's sake, a few more months, then they'd be alive today, and so you feel sad for those, but it really changed everything.

It was early July 1996, and the results of trials of combination therapy were being revealed at the IX International Conference on AIDS in Vancouver, Canada. Several presentations showed the powerful effects on progression of HIV infection, survival, and levels of HIV in the blood of people living with HIV (PLWH) (Williams and De Cock 1996). Thus began a new chapter in the treatment of HIV infection. Positive changes were in the air in terms of international efforts too. This was the year that UNAIDS, the Joint United Nations Programme on HIV/AIDS, started operations. Along with the World Health Organisation (WHO), UNAIDS developed joint initiatives with pharmaceutical companies to negotiate reduced prices for HIV drugs in developing countries (2000). The World Trade Organisation went on to announce the Doha Declaration, supporting the rights of developing countries to buy or manufacture generic HIV medications (2001). The Global Fund to Fight AIDS was established (2002), in 2003 PEPFAR, the US President's Emergency Plan for AIDS Relief was announced, and the Bill and Melinda Gates Foundation funded research on prevention.

In the UK, the introduction of effective antiretroviral therapies (ART) after 1996 started to have a significant impact on the morbidity and mortality of PLWH, although the number of new infections continued to increase. In 1996, there were 2,903 HIV and 1,468 AIDS diagnoses, with 1,481 HIV-related deaths, and by 2009, while the number of HIV diagnoses had increased to 6,630, AIDS diagnoses and HIV-related deaths had substantially declined, to 547 and 516 respectively (Health Protection Agency 2010). After 1996, the UK introduced antenatal testing for HIV amongst pregnant women, and those found to be positive were offered antiretroviral treatment, resulting in a greatly reduced risk of passing the infection to the baby. Medical and social services and charities would have to undergo considerable changes in subsequent years to adapt to the newly emerging HIV landscape. Funding continued to decline, while social attitudes towards HIV slowly became more accepting, albeit stigma persisted.

Is it really happening? Lazarus slowly

While 1996 is celebrated as the year when significant treatment advances were introduced, its benefits were not immediately obvious. There had already been too many false dawns, and it took some time for the sustained improvement in people's health to become apparent, and for hope to be realised, slowly, against a background of continuing losses. People living with HIV started to notice improvements in their health, but their descriptions of what was happening were couched in uncertainty. A PLWH recalled his early experience of the new treatments:

> I was one of the first to get the new treatments, people used to refer to the Lazarus effect, but Lazarus was brought back from the dead and walked, and it wasn't quite as sudden as that for me … the immune system slowly started to rebuild.

While in earlier years the choice was between one or two different antiretrovirals, gradually the alternatives involved different combinations of antiretrovirals. Perseverance, in spite of doubts, was typical of that early stage, and side-effects of the new treatments were often alarming, including visible signs, like facial wasting. Diarrhoea and mental health symptoms were not uncommon. Early combination therapies required large numbers of pills that came with strict guidance of how and when each should be taken. Adherence to medication was not easy, and failure led to an increase in viral load and subsequent treatment failure. Thus, the way events unfolded was less straightforward than the retrospective memory of success. And so, many PLWH kept trying one drug combination after another, and many continued to die. This heterosexual man referred to his slow and uncertain progress in response to the new treatments:

> The first combination I went on never worked, it brought the viral load down but not far enough. The second never worked for me, and it was only the third one that made my viral load undetectable … we didn't know how long it would last, and I was still unwell … and then very slowly I started getting better … they talked about the Lazarus effect, and it was Lazarus slowly … and one of the combination therapy side-effects was that it made you look worse, as you had facial wasting … there was never a eureka moment, it was incremental … I went to a lot of funerals after combination therapy came in.

Thus, treatment was not easy, and sceptical PLWH, like this man with haemophilia, had to go through their own fraught decision-making process to become convinced it was worth having a go at the new treatments:

> *They told me at the clinic about a combination therapy that was supposed to work well, but I said, oh don't be silly, this stupid treatment thing, it never works, you'll get really enthusiastic about it and then you look at the results and you go, well that didn't do anything … I then investigated and I read up about treatments and Vancouver, and I was stunned that it worked, so I thought, OK, well I'm obviously wrong there. So, I went back to the clinic and I said, OK I'll start the drugs.*

Professionals began to realise that although fewer people were seriously ill and dying, the number of people living with HIV continued to rise. However, the new treatments were not effective for everyone, especially when patients presented with advanced disease. What we were witnessing was a new world of pharmacological interventions and with information about the efficacy of treatments, drug interactions, and side-effects unfolding in real time, it took time for professionals to understand its complexities. Dangerous interactions between antiretrovirals and illicit drugs such as ecstasy (Henry and Hill 1998), and with complementary and alternative medicine substances (Stolbach et al. 2015), added to the need for clinicians and PLWH to become aware of the powerful effects of the new regimens. Additionally, to remain constructive to PLWH, clinicians had to alert PLWH about risks without judging their recreational drug use. A senior HIV physician who lived through the changing treatment scene talked about the new challenges faced by clinicians:

> *Nineteen ninety-six was the revolutionary moment, but of course that's much more retrospective. At the time we knew that treatment was improving greatly but we were still seeing people in very late disease who were still dying, who had inappropriate, less than perfect treatment. Although anti[retro]virals started in '96, '97, it wouldn't be until 2000 that you started to see quite a big change … a time of tremendous change in the drugs that were available, so we all had to become expert in drugs, in pharmacokinetics, in drug interactions, and adherence.*

Treatment adherence, and how to maintain it over the long term, became a crucial part of people's overall care. Pharmacists and clinical psychologists joined doctors and nurses in supporting PLWH to organise and manage their complex medical regimens. To ensure that adherence was kept at a very high level was regarded as paramount, and people were alerted to the fact that poor adherence was worse than not being on medication, as it was likely to increase viral resistance. The blunt message about the need for adherence was illustrated in this quote by a gay man living with HIV:

> *In those days [1998], because there were so few medications, adherence was the big thing. I was told, you are going to have to commit to this for the rest of your life. And so, the decisions were, we will bring you back into clinic for an appointment, but in the*

meanwhile we want you to think about everything and come back when you feel you can commit – it was, you are going to have to take pills morning and afternoon, and there may be side-effects etc, etc.

People working in HIV charities had similar mixed feelings of excitement and sadness, and a developing awareness of the changes ahead, as reported by a male charity worker:

In Vancouver the organisers were determined to have a good news story every day, that was my main memory, though a colleague was dying in London and we were getting daily updates about his health, and he died on the final day of the conference. So, there was this seismic change, but it had come too late for so many people … there was a lot of concern in case the drugs didn't work or stopped working after a certain amount of time, which was seen mostly in the AIDS specific wards, some of which had only just been completed. There had been massive investment in palliative care services too.

The development of new and effective treatments for HIV led activists to become intimately involved in understanding and publicising the more complex aspects of new treatments, such as their interactions and side-effects, as well as their efficacy, moving beyond their earlier efforts to provide practical and emotional support to PLWH. They helped to upskill and empower those affected by HIV in their interactions with doctors and researchers. Here is an example of active and critical involvement in the more detailed aspects of the new treatments by a gay man living with HIV:

I started combination therapy in '96, without any expectation of success, as I was a very late-stage person … so after that I became involved with community groups with people who had realised something was happening … there were community groups that were very much pro treatment, while other groups were against, treatments are poison, use as little as you want, and there were some doctors, including leading doctors, who really wanted to be cautious over treatment … I started following the research and following the data, and then started working with doctors who were excited to make it clear that something different was going on, so, that's when I started doing stuff more formally … we produced a newsletter that went out every two weeks by fax, because the field was changing so quickly.

At the same time as these treatment interventions were being implemented, prevention strategies applying psychological models of group behaviour aimed to change social normative behaviours about condom use. Latkin et al. (2010) argued for a slow diffusion of a model behaviour from a selected few to a target group. Key individuals within a peer group were educated in maintaining safe sexual behaviours, and taught how to promote them within their group, an approach that had proved successful in the US (Kelly et al. 1992), but less so in the UK (Kelly 2004).

Yes, it is happening! – The impact of the new antiretroviral therapies becomes clear

As PLWH started to respond to ART more positively, a change in the services they required became apparent. There was a reduction in the need for inpatient hospital care and an increase in demands for outpatient work. The changes in morbidity and mortality also had consequences for charities providing residential care and other services. Increasingly, living with – as opposed to dying with – HIV, also meant dealing with the psychological and social consequences of unexpected survival.

Impact on HIV hospital and community services

At the height of the HIV epidemic, specialist inpatient units were developed, with outpatient and day hospital facilities providing a comprehensive range of services, as discussed in earlier chapters. With successful combination therapy, HIV services had to be redesigned, and while the changes were welcome, as they reflected a better prognosis for people with HIV, they also forced a rethink on the way care was delivered. Changes were not always easy for our participants to accept, especially those directly involved in providing care. As a senior HIV nurse explained:

> The changes led to closure of wards and to redundancies, and some staff were very upset about the closures. And it's funny, isn't it? Because it was a good thing, but it was a terrible thing for us in other ways, but of course it was a good thing, people were getting well and not having to come in and they weren't so sick, but it did change a lot of things.

Sometimes the clinical changes that professionals and patients experienced were part of a wider reorganisation of services that was only indirectly linked to the need for changes in HIV care. The perceived outcomes, including the loss of HIV specialist wards and care teams, were mixed, as described by an HIV consultant:

> You won't be needing all these beds, they were saying, so we went to a situation where whenever you were admitted you were looked [after] for the duration of your stay by whoever you were admitted under … but these patients needed continuity.

Moving to a largely outpatient-based model of care also had implications for the work of nursing staff. Creative responses in some departments to the new care-demands led to a greater degree of teamwork and to an enhanced role for nursing staff, as described by a senior HIV nurse:

> The big task then was to look at the role of nursing, because they were getting loads more patients in, and they ended up just taking blood and doing observations and weighing patients, and their role became completely deskilled … so we tried to develop nurses as part of a multidisciplinary team but as independent practitioners … as it happened in diabetes, or cardiac conditions.

The work of community nurses diversified and became more complex, including not just home support and care of the dying, but also support for those experiencing serious medication side-effects, life-threatening co-morbidities, or mental health problems. As a community nurse said:

> *When combination therapy was introduced, district nurses were told that they would lose their jobs, but that didn't happen ... people with HIV were often very sick, either from treatment side-effects or from things like lymphoma or liver and kidney failure.*

Work on treatment adherence now became part of the job of the community nurses too, who, like the HIV physicians, had to develop new pharmacological skills:

> *I was supporting people through those really heavy pill burdens and the dietary requirements ... it was overwhelming for some people, especially young people who probably had never been ill before, never taken a pill before, to be faced with 30 odd pills a day was just shocking.*

Some PLWH, in particular those who injected drugs, experienced particular difficulties managing their medicines and clinic appointments, as illustrated by a psychiatric nurse:

> *I would go out and see people at home, and take their drugs to them at home. People couldn't organise themselves to get to the clinic, so I'd do bloods at home as well. I don't think I would be allowed to set up a service like that nowadays, there would be too many health and safety issues.*

Living with HIV

Chronic health problems, both HIV-related and unconnected, continued to affect the daily quality of life of PLWH, and mental health difficulties were common, often linked to social and financial problems. The possibility of returning to work, after many years away from it, was associated with self-doubt and concerns about a lack of skills, together with the difficulties involved in taking medication surreptitiously at regular intervals or taking time off to keep medical appointments. Relief at having survived for so long was tempered by a host of stresses and concerns. Keeping a sense of emotional balance while faced with such a mixture of difficulties and maintaining hope for the future felt to some like a full-time job. A gay man living with HIV commented on how tough the realities of living could be:

> *I wouldn't expect perfect health, and I think a lot of people who were very ill before the new treatments came but survived, have been damaged psychologically and physically ... so, that as well as the heart, the cancer and other things, I never got my life back together fully in the ways that most people would expect. There I was, living on disability benefits, in social housing, with no pension to look forward to, having not expected to live ... of course not expected to live and then living, but living much diminished in a sense.*

Not everybody acknowledged that significant changes had taken place. For some drug users, the stability achieved through treatment and survival was enough. Modest goals and acceptance of limited change were as necessary for those involved in helping people with addictions, as described by an experienced charity worker supporting injecting drug users (IDUs):

> *For people whose lives were a lot more chaotic, who were drug users, maybe still are drug users … sometimes not a lot has changed, it's just that they are alive. And maybe what we have been able to do, and the clinics have been able to do, is find small ways to make that more manageable.*

While over the years, gradually HIV treatment has become easier, with less demanding medication regimens and fewer side-effects, many still experience difficulties managing the complexity of hospital appointments. Unpleasant symptoms resulting from related infections, and adverse medication side-effects, remain a full-time job for many. A gay man living with HIV described the amount of planning involved:

> *The big challenge was clearly managing the medical side of things, we had appointments all over the place, so we had a big wall chart where we could see our appointments immediately and write down new ones. We managed the practical stuff pretty well, so that with diarrhoea, which I had and my partner suffered from too, we could deal with it effectively before leaving the house.*

The process of attempting to return to some form of normal living included having a sexual life again, something that had been a very important part of young lives in earlier days. Sex, in the context of HIV, brought back mixed memories of joy and loss. Restarting a sexual life was frequently complicated. News of the Swiss statement by HIV experts who, having reviewed the research evidence, argued that "PLWH on ART with completely suppressed viremia are not sexually infectious" (Vernazza et al. 2008), were immediately publicised in the UK HIV literature (Bernard 2008), adding a new element to the discussion of safer sex strategies. An HIV clinical psychologist talked about the changing picture:

> *When people were really sick, the last thing they felt like doing was having sex, so people weren't at risk of passing on the virus, but once you felt well you wanted sex again. So, a lot of prevention work started again … then we started to get news about how if you were on medication that reduced your viral load you were less likely to pass on the virus, so it led to more discussion about the need or otherwise for safer sex in a relationship.*

However, there remained a reluctance to promote this method of HIV prevention for some years. Only in 2011 did UK official guidance allude to the possibility that being on treatment might reduce people's infectiveness (NICE 2011). A man who has sex with men (MSM) living with HIV made an insightful comment early on:

> *In 2007 I went to the New and Emerging Prevention Technologies for Gay Men, and I thought, oh good … they will be talking about treatment. There was something about circumcision, about microbicides and about vaccines, so I thought right, chop off the end of your willy for a possible 60% reduction … [so I said], why aren't we talking about the prevention technology which will have a real impact, which is getting people to test and getting people on treatment, so they are un-infectious, and there were gasps of horror in the room.*

Resuming sexual activity was sometimes difficult, and sexual dysfunction problems, caused by a mixture of psychological and physical factors, became one of the new problems PLWH sought help for, as their health improved. A psychiatrist working with people with sexual dysfunction talked about some of the sexual difficulties that now needed to be addressed:

> *Treatment options were mostly limited to psychological treatments, which were seldom effective in PLWH, but in 1998 sildenafil (Viagra) became available in the US, and because it wasn't licensed in the UK, the hospital pharmacy was able to obtain it and we prescribed it on a 'named patient basis'. We prescribed carefully, as there were interactions with some of the antiretrovirals, and it was very effective … we developed a service so that patients would be assessed, and then a decision was made about whether medication or psychological treatment was appropriate. For many the problem wasn't sexual dysfunction, they were able to develop erections, but they were traumatised by the experience of coping with HIV, and they were terrified of relationships.*

Fear of transmitting HIV from a man to an uninfected female sexual partner while attempting to achieve pregnancy had left many couples childless. As ART restored many to good health and sperm washing was developed (a technique that enabled the virus to be removed from sperm), children became a possibility for such couples (Gilling-Smith 2000). A heterosexual man living with HIV described his experience:

> *When it looked like I was going to get well and I could have a normal lifespan, we had never had any children, and we thought maybe it would be possible … there was this process called sperm washing which would protect my wife from being infected.*

Very few clinics offered this service, and when additional fertility problems occurred, there were only a few private fertility clinics who would accept PLWH (Balet et al. 1998). The heterosexual man quoted earlier expressed his disappointment:

> *If it was any other area of medicine that involved the majority of HIV-positive people, they wouldn't get away with it. Fertility clinics in the UK do not accept HIV-positive people.*

HIV family services for pregnant women with HIV required both professional cooperation and utmost sensitivity. A paediatrician involved in the care of HIV infected babies and young children outlined some of the steps taken to ensure good collaboration between mothers and teams:

> *Following referral from the obstetrician or a midwife of a woman identified to have HIV, after we had antenatal screening in 1999, I would make contact, meet the mother, explain the nature of the follow up, about the very intensive visits, taking blood, antibiotics for the first six weeks of the baby's life before we knew whether the child was infected, and how important it was not to breastfeed … Once the baby was born, I would then get a call from the maternity hospital, and we would start the follow ups, and it made it easier that you've met the woman antenatally.*

Family-centred models of care which had been set up in earlier years were further developed to provide care not only to affected parents and children, but widened their scope to include the foster parent when needed, as described by an HIV paediatrician:

> *Many of these infected children were either adopted or in long-term foster care, and the people who had fostered them always said, we must tell the children, because the foster carers had nothing to lose, you can talk to the child about why you have HIV, it doesn't reflect badly on you, but if the child's mother is a street worker and a drug user, it is a bit difficult if the child asked, how did I get my HIV, how did you get it, Mum? It was very emotional for the birth mothers to disclose the diagnosis.*

Impact on mental health provision

As the prognosis of living with HIV began to change, PLWH encountered new psychological and social difficulties. The focus of their concerns shifted from dealing with serious illness and likely death, to having to face the prospect, uncertain as it was at first, but which would turn out to be a much-extended life span.

At the same time, a number of studies were suggesting an association between the acquisition of HIV and mental health problems, particularly depression, bipolar disorder, and alcohol and substance misuse, as well as risky sexual behaviour (Carey et al. 2004; Meade et al. 2008), indicating the importance of continuing to provide interventions to support individuals in modifying behaviours associated with an increased risk of transmission. Motivational interviewing approaches together with cognitive-behavioural skills training were used to promote safer sex and drug use (Rietmeijer et al. 1996), although the efficacy of these approaches was difficult to evaluate due to the typically small studies and selected participants.

The majority of HIV units had links with the local mental health services, often having their own mental health professionals attached to the service. In many large teams, the appointment of psychiatric nurses to support PLWH receiving treatment in the general hospital had been a development for some time, and their role broadened and strengthened as the epidemic evolved post-96, as described by one such female psychiatric nurse:

> *I was a member of the HIV multidisciplinary team and also of the mental health liaison service, and I had a lot of contact with the psychiatrists and involved [them] when I needed them. But it changed a lot over time. When I first started there in 1998, combination therapy had only been around for a couple of years and already was making a big difference. Most of the people I saw were severely mentally ill, and it was about arranging Mental Health Act assessments, most of them with no history of mental health problems before HIV, but with problems as a result of living with HIV, either the psychological fallout of it, or actual psychiatric illness from it.*

Some HIV services, like those that served a large population of injecting drug users, developed flexible ways of working, ensuring that PLWH remained engaged with the service, which included counsellors and clinical psychologists, and dealt with a range of HIV-related and also pre-existing disorders. A psychiatrist working in such a setting described her work:

> *I had wondered whether I would only deal with HIV-related problems, but I soon realised there was an equal need amongst those with mild or moderate unrelated mental health problems, so I would say I was working with HIV mental health patients. Our team offered flexibility in terms of seeing patients at home as well as in the clinic. This is a good model, especially from the nurses' side – for some patients home visits are the only contact, and the nurses would do blood tests and deliver antiretrovirals too, while monitoring mental health.*

Doctors working with PLWH and injecting drug users had to reset their goals and management of addiction, even when the changes of success were limited:

> *We had this paradoxical reaction where everybody just said, well I'm not dying but I'm dying. We said, no you're not dying. But people had got it into their minds that they were dying, and there was an adjustment to people's lives and in terms of prescribing. We'd set ourselves on this course of palliative care, and were giving people 200 mg of methadone, and some chlorpromazine, and some whatever else they wanted, some morphine if they wanted it, and plenty of Valium. And all of a sudden, we had to say, oh well we can't go on doing this.*

Acute psychiatric problems, such as psychoses and acute brain syndromes, became less common as the new treatments became established. PLWH now faced the prospect of chronic, longer-term mental health difficulties, associated with the confirmation that they were now more likely to survive than not (Adams et al. 2016). An HIV psychiatrist described some of these changes:

> *There was less of a need for inpatient psychiatric work, as the [medical] inpatient beds started to close, it was mostly outpatient work. The HIV doctors had very busy clinics, and so the mental health team developed outpatient clinics with psychiatrists, psychologists, and the psychiatric nurse, who was embedded in the HIV clinical team. We were seeing many PLWH who had long-term difficulties, often manifesting as depression, a diagnosis that became more common.*

Impact on HIV charities

HIV charities had played a fundamental role from the start of the epidemic in the UK, providing a wide range of services for PLWH and those affected by HIV. They included emotional and practical support and counselling, as well as residential care, both respite and end of life, and work on prevention and education. As was the case for HIV clinical care, the need for charity involvement changed significantly with the success of combination therapy. Local authority funding was less accessible, and resources tended to be made more available to the larger charities. Funding changes became an important factor in the reorganisation of charities. As end of life care facilities became less necessary, the focus shifted towards provision of services for those with chronic difficulties, such as HIV brain-related conditions and convalescent care. Charities providing counselling and support who had provided help for those ill and dying, started to shift their focus towards support for living, such as providing benefits advice, and assistance for a return to employment. Some of these changes were seen as inevitable and, perhaps, even desirable, as funding prioritised the need for effective medications. A gay man, an activist who was also living with HIV, commented on the impending changes:

> In the '90s, the government was pouring money into organisations supporting people with HIV because there was nothing else, they didn't have any medicines that worked, so they might as well pay you to go on holidays to swim with a dolphin, to give an actual example I benefited from. But later the money had to go into the pills, and there are people saying silly things like, oh it got medicalised. Of course, it got bloody medicalised, the pills started working, that's how you cure people, so I understand where the money had to go … I'm not surprised that a lot of money that had gone into support went out of it.

A senior charity worker expressed his concern about the impact of the changes resulting from both the focus on medical treatments and the increasing financial pressures. Highlighting the role of the voluntary sector in the development of innovative forms of care, often ahead of the statutory sector, he talked about the weakening and loss of integration between sectors that was becoming apparent now:

> It's very traditional that when new ground is being broken, it's often broken in the voluntary sector before the statutory sector gets it and embraces it, and I think that's what happened. I think our whole concept of the integrated model and continuum of care and services slotting together was ahead of where the statutory sector was then … the challenges for us didn't come until the mid '90s, when the focus went from care to treatment, and the money too.

Other factors, however, linked to the epidemiological changes affecting the HIV population in the UK, were also important in altering the needs of PLWH accessing charities, and adding to the uncertainty. The evolution of the London

Lighthouse, an iconic and very influential charity providing residential palliative care services and support (Cantacuzino 1993; Spence 1996), illustrates clearly the changing picture. Services that had provided for a primarily MSM population, now had to respond to the needs of other groups, such as women and families, and African PLWH. A nurse working in a charity service referred to some of these changes:

> *The patients at the residential unit were changing. It had initially been pretty much all gay men and IV drug users. The needle exchange programmes came in very quickly in the '80s, and so the IV drug-using population was dropping off very quickly. New drug users weren't getting infected, it was the old ones that had shared needles because there were no other options ... we were getting more African patients, so there was a change in population. And I don't think it was because there were more of them, I think it was because we became more accessible to them ... there was conflict also between the de-gaying of the charity and making it more accessible to women ... the two main groups using the charity had different needs. Most of the women who were IV drug users didn't have kids or if they had, they were in care ... but a lot of the African women who were using the service had kids, and the childcare services for mothers and children carried on a lot longer than the residential unit.*

The demise of the residential unit and eventually, the charity, was symptomatic of the changing circumstances, with a much-reduced need for palliative care beds, and a harbinger of further shifts in care provision:

> *The charity was an interesting place, it started when the death rate was pretty high, and a lot of people chose to die there because they were cared for and well supported, and it was a preferable choice to dying at home. And it is really sad because first, it was sold to another charity in 2000 and the residential unit closed and became supported housing flats, but the ground floor was used for drop-in HIV services and different therapies, until it finally closed a couple of years ago.*

As highlighted previously, the expected high prevalence of an HIV-dementia, or AIDS Dementia Complex, anticipated by earlier research (Navia et al. 1986), never materialised (Catalan and Thornton 1993), and the introduction of combination therapies made the syndrome even less likely, although at the time there were still PLWH needing high levels of care for other brain-related disorders. Nevertheless, funding problems led to the closure of community-based facilities, such as Patrick House in London, and there were consequences. A nurse working in the charity sector described some unwelcome outcomes of these developments:

> *They had severe cognitive impairment or dementia, or severe mental health problems, a good half had drug and alcohol related issues, and they couldn't function on a daily basis ... once a person was accepted, they were there until the end of their life, and because it was such a small household, when somebody died it really affected everybody ... when Princess Diana died in 1997, there was a lot of trauma, people were irrationally upset, and three months later we were told we were closing, we weren't told why but I felt they'd lost a tender ... it was a shame. We had to rehouse or move people on ... I know*

of one person who went to sheltered housing but then died because he left the iron on the ironing board and that set the flat on fire … that should never have happened.

Some charities survived by adapting to the changing circumstances, developing new roles and merging with other organisations providing similar services. As the epidemiology of HIV changed, services for women and children, and for asylum seekers and non-gay PLWH, became more pressing, and the charity sector had to adapt to increasingly complex presentations, as shown by the experience of an HIV charity worker:

> *Previously the charity had been for white gay men and a few drug users, and then suddenly there was an influx of Black Africans, so managing that was quite interesting in the sense of how people saw other people with HIV, how they saw the charity changing. Suddenly we needed to start thinking about women's services because obviously the majority of African clients were women. We need to start thinking about kids' stuff and had to start thinking about extreme poverty … Some left because they didn't like it, but many more came in and we managed that successfully, and we helped integrate the asylum seekers there who had HIV, so that worked quite well.*

Redeveloping the services provided by HIV charities, against a backdrop of funding restrictions and changing needs, was not an easy task. There was an understandable resistance to change both amongst users of the services and those working with the charities. Nevertheless, difficult choices had to be made to fit within reduced budgets. A senior charity worker describes the turmoil faced by charity services:

> *We realised things were going to change, and some might get very attached to the services they had been used to … we also knew that we were likely to see funding reduced for social care and for broader social support, and probably for HIV prevention as well … it actually meant that a number of these services were going to have to close … by merging we could reduce the infrastructure costs, one chief executive instead of two and one auditor instead of two, and so on, and redirect those savings either into service delivery or in managing the impact of cuts … the whole period of redesigning services, closing some down, opening others up in an era of self-management was both immensely challenging and immensely rewarding.*

Balancing models of care: from person-centred to medication-based care

The relationship between PLWH and those providing care and support also underwent changes. When treatment interventions were limited and there was there was little that could be effectively done to treat HIV, medical and psychosocial interventions aimed to minimise the impact of symptoms, disability, and social adversity. Under these circumstances, the person living with HIV had come to be at the centre of well-coordinated efforts of a multidisciplinary team, and relationships between carers and PLWH had become close and informal.

The closeness of the relationship between PLWH and their carers became apparent in the case of some forms of treatment, such as the cosmetic treatment of facial wasting. Side-effects of the new combination therapies included this stigmatising manifestation of illness that could signal to the world the nature of the person's diagnosis. A specialist nurse who administered the treatment described the intimate communication involved in her relationship with PLWH:

> *I started treating facial wasting in 2001. Treating facial wasting was very powerful. I think it was because we did it in private, but also because you're touching somebody's face, and a lot of the people that I treated hadn't had their faces touched for a long time, and we forget how intimate touching a face is. Your mother touches your face, your lover touches your face. And if you feel that you are wearing the virus on your face, people don't touch you. And so suddenly I was touching people's faces, I was in their body space, and it was every intimate ... and they sat down and often talked and talked, because there was a lot that they needed to say and that they needed somebody to hear ... and then when they go away you almost want to shed a tear, but are you shedding a tear because of them, or because they've come into your day?*

As the introduction of new and effective treatment gathered pace, the focus of interventions and care changed, shifting towards managing medications. This sometimes came at the expense of managing the condition in partnership with PLWH, as had been the case previously. Here, an HIV physician and a PLWH reflect on this change, suggesting that the traditional medical approach had become more central again, with some loss of the person-centred model. The HIV physician referred to the changes with some feeling of regret:

> *The drugs were pretty difficult to take long term, there were lots of toxicities and adherence problems, and once you've got them working, you can shift to side-effects and how to minimise them ... so there was a big shift away from the patient being at the centre of care to the drugs being at the centre.*

This PLWH enlarged on the physician's feelings of regret with his added critical comments on the context of social and political developments:

> *We had a good model of care, and then in '96 when the effective polypharmacy came through, that's when the old attitude resurfaced, and physicians said, oh we're in charge now, at the same time as the community lost its ability to know what to do, because the crisis wasn't there anymore ... well the crisis is still here, but it had reduced and so you got this separation and this fractionation again, and then the recreation of silos, against an economic context of increasing neoliberalism which was also about managerialism and atomisation ... the services had got there in terms of inpatient care and hospice care, but not so much in outpatient care because that was considered to be specialist care.*

The shift towards a more medical management model was uncomfortable for some, who feared it represented a return to an outdated approach, one characterised by a 'doctor-knows-best' attitude, far from the purposive empowerment of PLWH which was apparent in the early days of the epidemic, as stated by a gay man living with HIV:

> *The problem is the physician-centred culture, so one of the solutions is to create models that learned from the best of what existed previously, and also is involvement with the community … you will only create real impact if you've got empowered people with the condition who are your anchors to the response.*

This view was not universally supported, however, and other PLWH who had been living with HIV for many years, spoke up about the ongoing strength and equality of their patient–doctor relationship. This alliance had not appeared to them to have been affected by the availability of new treatments, perhaps unlike newer partnerships. Here are the views of a man who had been living with HIV for many decades:

> *My HIV doctor hasn't treated me in a doctor–patient kind of relationship that I imagine most people have, a doctor–patient relationship where the patients think that the doctor is a god, and I don't subscribe to that at all, and she doesn't subscribe to it either. I think a lot of HIV patients had this kind of relationship with their clinicians, and I think the further you go back the more you realise the partnership.*

Sharing the experience of learning about the new treatments became an element in the original partnership between PLWH and their professional carers. This partnership had its roots in the earlier advent of gay liberation which had politicised gay rights and communities at the time when HIV had first appeared. A heterosexual man living with HIV provided some context to the evolution of the relationships between patients and doctors:

> *My relationship with my doctor was one of equality. After the Vancouver conference, we're all starting from the same base point. At the start of it, I couldn't read a research paper, at the end of it I can read a research paper, and that's the same as what my HIV doctor could do. So we learnt at the same time to a certain extent. There was a complete breakdown of the normal, 'yes doctor, please doctor' thing. Our cohort was unusual, you got relatively young, educated men, and because of that, people were bolshie and the gay men were used to campaigning around human rights, so that was incredibly helpful, and I stand on the shoulders of the many men that campaigned and fought for access to treatment, and lots of other straight people who fought for it as well.*

When there were limited treatment options available, personal involvement in decision making and evaluation of the needs of the person living with HIV was the rule for many HIV physicians, rather than a standard approach focused on medication concerns. After the successful introduction of ART, some physicians tended to perceive some of their HIV patients as having fewer specific needs, and thus only needing to be managed in a more traditional way, comparable to the management of people suffering from non-HIV-related chronic conditions. However, many patients continued to require a good deal of involvement and care, that often focused on treatment adherence. A senior HIV physician recognised a significant shift in the pattern of care provided about 10 years after the introduction of effective ART:

> It's probably not until 2006/07 that there is a dramatic change. The drugs became once or twice a day, really very easy to tolerate, with relatively few side-effects. So the population attending clinics changes because it becomes people who have very disordered lives and therefore can't take the pills on a regular basis so drug users, recreational and others, become much more important, alcoholics become much more important, and people with psychological difficulties who couldn't take the pills. As a group you spend much more time dealing with them. The average guy without problems, able to take the pills, you could see once or twice a year.

As treatment adherence became a major concern, both charities and statutory services developed programmes to support PLWH who had difficulties taking their medication regularly, especially at the outset, when treatment regimens were very complex, involving multiple tablets, timing issues, and strict adherence regimes. Charities, in particular, found a new role in facilitating HIV peer support group and individual assistance that focused on helping PLWH maintain good treatment adherence. A charity worker explained some of the changes:

> A particular service that hadn't been part of our brief until now was adherence. Between '96 and, what, 2005, the number of potential combinations grew and grew, and then became clear which the winners were, which worked and crucially, which could be manufactured together in the same pill, and so move to one pill a day. The range of choices and the number of decisions both clinicians and people with HIV had to make is no longer an issue, but for a considerable period of time it really was.

Mission accomplished?

Towards the end of the first decade of the new century there was a general sense that HIV had been sorted. HIV seldom made the UK media headlines, or when it did, it was to emphasise how HIV was now a chronic, manageable disease. Now all seemed well with PLWH. Mortality and morbidity had certainly showed remarkable improvements, but there were still many issues to resolve.

The perception of PLWH and their professional carers of what it was like to be now living with HIV was more nuanced. They acknowledged the progress made in terms of survival, but identified many unresolved issues which needed to be faced. Activists and charity workers recognised the changes that had taken place and that many of the original goals had been achieved. For many, this was a time to rethink their involvement and commitment. Similarly, for professionals that had spent, in some cases, several decades closely engaged in dealing with HIV and its consequences, this was a time to review their roles.

Laying down their arms

Charity workers and activists, many of whom had spent years battling to develop and maintain services, at times against major political and financial obstacles, were starting to feel that most objectives had been achieved. They were also ready to acknowledge their exhaustion, as a senior charity worker clearly described:

> *After 10 years I felt I'd done all that I could do, and I didn't necessarily want to do that for the rest of my life, and that time was up. I was exhausted after 10 years and ready. At the time I would have told you I was very well supported but thinking about what I do now with my mentoring, I don't think there was much support. There were large numbers of very generous and kind supporters and there were a few people who were personally very supportive, but I think the whole thing did take its toll. Partly it was all a bit in the glare of a lot of publicity, and I'm an introvert, so I was going against type a lot to do the job.*

Adjusting to surviving without having constantly to fight and engage in HIV activism when most goals had been seemingly achieved, led some PLWH to a sense of aimlessness and loss of identity. There was a search for new life objectives, a position made very explicit by some charity workers and activists, like this gay man living with HIV:

> *And then combination therapy came along and completely messed up the plan. And it was extraordinarily difficult to readjust to, having thought, OK, I've done the best with my life, now I'm ready to go, and I accept what's going to happen, and I've done whatever planning I need to do, and then to think that none of that applied anymore. What on earth am I going to do? I haven't done anything for ten years apart from AIDS activism. I don't know anything else now, I don't have a career. I had been cutting myself off from an awful lot of things that had given me an identity. What do I do now? I got myself mentally retired and I thought, shall I try and start a new career? … So in 2004 I decided with my partner to move to the countryside where I live now, which was still part and parcel of thinking this is what retirement is … but it is difficult being happy when you've known a time in your life where it's been so intense with having to do things and get things done, and having to achieve things that are sedentary, life without goals, really.*

In the UK, many HIV charities experienced a loss of volunteers and activists who had been involved for some years. The lack of a sense of crisis and urgency had made UK-based work less special and unique, as this charity worker explains:

> *What it also did, was it allowed a lot of people who had been volunteering in the sector to leave and to go off and do other things, and that was unexpected but a number of people by 1998/1999, were saying to us, I've done this for 5, 8, 10 years, and I want to go and do something different now, there's continued transmission, but people aren't dying in the numbers that they were, things are getting better … It also allowed a new cadre of people to come in as well, and it was quite a surprise to me. It happened, to a degree, with nursing*

staff, less so amongst doctors. It changed the uniqueness and the importance of doing AIDS work. It became less of [a] social and less of a professional cache quite rapidly after that.

As in the case of charity workers, new professional carers who had not worked through the years of serious illness and death, when there seemed to be no effective treatments but relationships between professional carers and PLWH were close and empathetic, did not necessarily appreciate those more egalitarian interactions. The change of attitude amongst nursing staff was certainly recognised by this gay man living with HIV, who identified a loss of personal involvement and expertise, and who missed the degree of closeness that as a long-term patient he had previously experienced:

A lot of nurses at the time were so used to being so heavily involved with their patients. It wasn't just about medicines, it was caring in the Florence Nightingale sense of being a nurse, if that makes sense? You were dealing with people who were dying, you dealt with people who the nurses used to help take out of hospital so that they could die at home … these were people who were going to funerals, and these were people for whom we were not patients, we were much more than patients. And gradually, as things started to get better for HIV-positive people and the medicine started to come on board, that level of intensity, that level of knowledge, that level of experience, and for nurses in this whole partnership model where they weren't just a nurse, they were kind of specialists in their own right. And I guess what happened was that they got bored and thought, I'm a bit bored now because sticking needles into somebody and giving their obs every 15 minutes is boring compared to what I used to do. And so, what you see is a turnover of staff and they don't have the same approach.

There was less of a changeover of senior doctors, but when it happened, the sense of loss amongst PLWH could be hard to take, in particular for those having received HIV care for decades. This Black Afro-Caribbean female nurse talked about a kind of abandonment experienced by PLWH that might have seemed unimaginable in the early days of the epidemic:

Patients talk about their doctors, whom they have been seeing for years, and now the doctors are retiring and dying, and they never thought they would see their doctors retire … we were telling them that they were going to leave us, and in fact, we are leaving them. They do feel a sense of bereavement.

Struggling to continue

The success of combination therapy brought about major changes for PLWH, which were only gradual from 1996, but culminated in significant change, not only for PLWH, but also for their professional carers, health services, and charities. The person-centred model of care that had developed in earlier times, when treatment options were limited and of minimal effectiveness, was put under pressure. The focus of care moved towards managing medication and its technical and practical aspects. The person-centred model did survive in some ways, even if currents were flowing in a different, more medical direction. For some, it felt as if HIV care was returning to a traditional model of care, partly as result of focus on pharmacological treatment, but also due to the wider political changes. While for the media and public discourse HIV had by now ceased to be a problem, on the ground difficulties continued, with many PLWH continuing to struggle with their physical health and psychological difficulties.

Against this background there were indications that, in spite of ongoing social and political difficulties, positive new developments concerning the prevention of HIV transmission were giving hope to the possibility of eradicating HIV infection once and for all.

References

Adams C, Zacharia S, Masters L, Coffey C and Catalan P (2016) Mental health problems in PLWH: changes in the last two decades 1990–2014. *AIDS Care*, 28(S1), 56–59.

Balet R, Lower A, Wilson C, Anderson J and Grudzinskas J (1998) Attitudes towards routine HIV screening and fertility treatment in HIV positive patients – a survey. *Human Reproduction (Oxford, England)*, 13(4), 1085–1087.

Bernard E (2008) Swiss experts say individuals with undetectable viral load and no STI cannot transmit HIV during sex. *NAM aidsmap*, 30 January 2008. London, NAM Publications.

Cantacuzino M (1993) *Till Break of Day*. London, Heineman.

Carey MP, Carey KB, Maisto SA, Schroder KE, Vanable PA, Gordon CM (2004) HIV risk behavior psychiatric outpatients: association with psychiatric disorder, substance use disorder, and gender. *The Journal of Nervous and Mental Disease*, 192(4), 289.

Catalan J and Thornton S (1993) Whatever happened to HIV-associated dementia? *International Journal of STD and AIDS*, 4, 1–4.

Gilling-Smith C (2000) HIV prevention: Assisted reproduction in HIV discordant couples. *The AIDS Reader*, 10(10), 581–587.

Health Protection Agency (2010) http://www.hpa.org.uk/web/HPAweb&HPAwebStandard /HPweb_C/1203496957984

Henry JA and Hill R (1998) Fatal interaction between ritonavir and MDMA. *The Lancet*, 352, 1751–1752.

Kelly JA (2004) Popular opinion leaders and HIV prevention peer education: resolving discrepant findings, and implications for the development of effective community programmes. *AIDS Care*, 16(2), 139–150.

Kelly JA, St Lawrence JS, Stevenson LY, Hauth AC, Kalichman SC, Diaz YE and Morgan MG (1992) Community AIDS/HIV risk reduction: the effects of endorsements by popular people in three cities. *America Journal of Public Health*, 82(11), 1483–1489.

Latkin C, Weeks MR, Glasman L, Galletly C and Albarracin D (2010) A dynamic social systems model for considering structural factors in HIV prevention and detection. *AIDS and Behavior*, 14(2), 222–238.

Meade CS, Graff FS, Griffin ML and Weiss RD (2008) HIV risk behaviour among patients with co-occurring bipolar and substance use disorders: associations with mania and drug abuse. *Drug and Alcohol Dependence*, 92(1–3), 296–300.

Navia BA, Jordan BD and Price RW (1986) The AIDS dementia complex: I clinical features. *Annals of Neurology*, 19, 517–524.

NICE (2011) *NICE Public Health Guidance 34: Increasing the uptake of HIV testing to reduce undiagnosed infection and prevent transmission among men that have sex with men*. London, National Institute for Health and Clinical Excellence.

Rietmeijer CA, Kane MS, Simons P, Corby NH, Wolitski RJ, and Cohn DL (1996) Increasing the use of bleach and condoms among injecting drug users in Denver: outcomes of a targeted, community level HIV prevention program. *AIDS*, 10(3), 291–298.

Spence C (1996) *On Watch: Views from the Lighthouse*. London, Cassell.

Stolbach A, Paziana K, Heverling H and Pham P (2015) A review of toxicity of HIV medications II: Interactions with drugs and complementary and alternative medicine products. *Journal of Medical Toxicology*, 11 (3): 326–341.

Vernazza P, Hirschel B, Bernasconi E, and Flepp M(2008) Les personnes seropositsives ne souffrant d'aucune autre MST et suivant un traitment antiretroviral efficace ne transmettent pas le VIH par voie sexuelle. *Bulletin des Medecines Suisses*, 89 (5) 165–169.

Williams IG and De Cock KM (1996) The IX International Conference on AIDS Vancouver 7–12 July 1996. A review of Clinical Science Track B. *Genitourinary Medicine*, 72: 365–369.

5 They think it's all over: 'It's just a chronic illness'

Introduction

The idea that living with HIV infection is akin to having a chronic illness has become a common rhetoric in medicine. While the notion contains a significant element of truth, it also underestimates the impact of HIV on the lives of people living with HIV (PLWH). HIV is, in fact, not an easily manageable chronic condition, but one that is frequently associated with difficult co-morbidities. It is also a condition that is still linked to considerable levels of stigma, anxiety, and fear. Additionally, it is a condition that continues disproportionately to affect populations already facing economic and social disadvantage and discrimination (HIV Psychosocial Network 2018).

In 2008, the international financial crash brought the global economic system close to the edge of collapse. In the ensuing political upheaval, by 2010 a newly elected coalition government of the Conservative and Liberal Democrat parties was formed in the UK, with a promise of implementing financial austerity. This policy saw the introduction of 20% public spending budget cuts over the next four years. Additionally, after the 2016 EU referendum, the complex process of negotiating the UK's exit from the EU led to the neglect of non-Brexit related political and social issues, including those concerning health and social care.

Changes in the provision of statutory health and care services, including the reduction in the number of inpatient and palliative care beds available, and the role and extent of the work of HIV charities, were also significant. Some of the changes were understandable as a result of the changing picture of HIV, with reductions in morbidity and mortality. The number of new HIV diagnoses in the UK fell from 6,327 in 2010 to 4,363 in 2017, and from 718 to 428 deaths respectively (Public Health England 2017a). Other changes in funding and provision of services were more motivated by political ideology, in what Squire (2013, p182–185) has described as "the narratives of marketization of HIV", reflecting a broader fragmentation of NHS care. Here, the impact of the Health and Social Care Act of 2012 in England and Wales (the Lansley reforms introduced by the coalition government), are being felt now. Care and prevention for HIV are now separated into different commissioning and funding streams, leading to a fragmentation of services.

Sexual health budgets (which local authorities in post-Lansley England are responsible for), have been reduced in most local authorities, with an estimated reduction
in funding for non-clinical services for HIV of 28% from 2015–16 to 2016–17
(White 2017). Serious discussion of the future of HIV services in the NHS has
started (Baylis et al. 2017; NAT 2016).

In parallel with these changes, came a resurgence of interest in the prevention
of new HIV infections, the result of two important research and policy developments.
First, confirmation that effective antiretroviral treatment of HIV leads to the bodily
fluids of an infected person becoming non-infectious (Vernazza et al. 2008),
making knowledge of HIV status and early, effective treatment imperative in
preventing onward transmission. In 2014, the Joint United Nations Programme on
HIV/AIDS (UNAIDS) launched the 90–90–90 targets, aiming at 90% of PLWH
to be diagnosed, 90% of those diagnosed to be accessing antiretroviral treatment,
and 90% of those accessing treatment to achieve viral suppression by 2020.
Organisations around the world (NAM 2017) endorsed in 2017 the "Undetectable
= Untransmittable" (U=U) motto (UNAIDS 2018). Second, evidence for the
preventive role of post-exposure prophylaxis (PEP) (Siedner, Tumarkin, and
Bogoch, 2018) and pre-exposure prophylaxis (PrEP) gathered momentum as the
decade continued (Grant, Lama, Anderson et al., 2010; McCormack, Dunn, Desai
et al., 2016). The growing evidence for treatment-related prevention led to a
resurgence of activism, involving community action in collaboration with clinicians
and researchers, aiming to make treatment more widely acceptable and freely
available on the NHS.

Living with HIV now: not bad but not always good

Following the introduction of effective antiretroviral therapy (ART), which initially involved a complex regimen of medications, progress was made in the development of once a day therapy or fixed-dose combinations combining two or three
drugs in one pill. This approach which by now was routinely recommended
(BHIVA 2003), showed a significant effect in enhancing treatment adherence
(Bangalore et al. 2007). For some PLWH, the experience of living and struggling
for many years with HIV has had complex outcomes. Coming to terms with their
feelings about HIV itself, many PLWH's own feelings about themselves, and their
encounters with contemporary public attitudes, have resulted in a sense of self-
acceptance and gratitude. There is a recognition of the value of the help they
received, as described both by this Black African woman and by a gay man:

> *I think without HIV I might have taken life for granted. I know it's a real gift, especially
> given that I still have it, when a lot of people in my situation have long gone. It makes
> you be thankful for every day you wake up and you are well. Nor do I take the HIV
> services for granted.*

> *I consider myself on the whole extremely fortunate, and I'm alive, I'm in love, I've had
> some very good people at the hospitals, I've had very good care, I've just been very lucky.*

HIV has ceased to be a problem for some. A hint of gallows humour is present in this account by a man with haemophilia and HIV of his current state of health, and of his likely future health problems:

> *I have haemophilia problems, my joints are wearing out, but they have to last until I die, which I think is going to be early '70s, because that seems to be when haemophiliacs die. The nice thing about haemophiliacs is that now we mainly die of bleeding, we have gone back to where we were before HIV and hepatitis came along, it's our proper haemophilia that's causing us problems and killing us.*

The experience of living with HIV is not always positive, however. For many PLWH now, current difficulties and co-morbidities, such as heart disease, associated cancers, or gastrointestinal problems, and concerns about the future, colour their living experience. A former injecting drug user (IDU) describes her daily problems coping with life, not helped by her worries about her future health unrelated to HIV:

> *My memory is really bad, I forget to take my pills. My son texts me every morning, Mum, take your pills. I still don't take them, I forget that he has texted me. In the last five years I have lost a lot of people but not to HIV, they've died of cancer. So, I am starting to think, this is me, you are venturing out into something new and unknown and that's your future, because something you never contemplated was actually having that future.*

HIV is not just a chronic treatable disease, multiple factors influence responses to the condition, some being part of the baggage acquired before HIV, and others that come along with the infection, or will declare themselves in the future. For instance, past bereavements and anticipated losses add to the difficulties coping with haemophilia for this PLWH:

> *I find it hard to feel very much more optimistic about my future health, partly because my arthritic problems have been worse … the feeling of mortality is with me for all sort of reasons, maybe it's my wife's illness, my brother's death, haemophiliacs with HIV who have died, and my parents, and so, yes, bereavement is a big part of my mental life.*

Health workers in the community recognise the increasing complexity of the lives of the people they are trying to support at home, away from consultations in large HIV clinics. They see PLWH attempting to cope with multiple complex problems, all against a background of cuts to social services, with care now being carried out by agency workers who cannot be expected to manage such complicated issues. A male community nurse described the current situation:

> *Every patient I have now, as opposed to when I started when you had PLWH who were fairly stable but needed just somebody to encourage them with their medication, nearly everybody now has 30 different complexities, not just HIV which is very low*

down on that list. Their housing is terrible, they are awaiting three departments to get their act together to get them in for rehab, or surgery. And the quality of the home carers is very poor, don't know how to manage their HIV medication, are not there for long, and a lot of them don't really speak English well. My patients who have carers have been through two or three agencies to try and find somebody who would fit.

Being alive now, an unexpected success for some long-term survivors, is also a mixed blessing. Many now see themselves as forgotten, struggling to adapt to their limited life opportunities, in addition to having regularly to justify their reliance on benefits. A female Black Afro-Caribbean nurse outlined the plight of some of her patients:

They were diagnosed in their 20s, and were told they weren't going to live for long, they didn't think they'd see their 30s, but they did. They didn't think they would see their 40s, but they did. They are in their 50s and some approaching their 60s, and ageing is very difficult for them. And where do you pick up? Their benefits have been stopped, they are told they have to get back to work, it's a bit like I've suddenly got to learn a new language, and I've got to learn it very quickly.

The experience of PLWH diagnosed in the ART era shows an interesting range of responses. Research from the Netherlands, focusing on the HIV-related burden of people diagnosed between 2014 and 2018, described an early stage of 'medicalisation' of life (pill taking, medical appointments) and distressing emotions linked to the shock of diagnosis, which subsequently declined over time, only to be followed up with the emergence of more persistent concerns about stigma, disclosure, and sexual lives (Bilsen 2019).

Stigma is still with us

"*Just because it's changed, just because its face has changed doesn't mean to say that it's a disease without stigma, is it? Is it? I don't think so, I don't think so,*" stated a female Black Afro-Caribbean nurse.

The fact that HIV infection is not associated as frequently as before with physical health changes and an altered appearance means that PLWH can avoid having to disclose their status. Paradoxically, while being able to 'pass' can sometimes be protective, it can also lead to problems such as isolation, and a dangerous pretence that all is well when it is not. A charity worker commented on these changes brough about by ART:

AIDS was very visible, HIV is not, and that brings us back to the problem of disclosure. In the past, people with AIDS had no choice … some people tried to dress it up as cancer or other disease … the lack of disclosure means for many that they don't know anybody with HIV, and the smaller their support network becomes.

PLWH from communities already facing discrimination on ethnic and economic grounds, such as Black and other ethnic minority groups, experience a double burden of stigma when HIV is added to the mix. The situation was described by a Black African support worker in relation to the difficulties Black African people can have when being more open and disclosing HIV:

> Last week I went to visit a support group of mostly African people, and I met a man who knew about the group for over a year, but had never had the courage to attend, and when he actually came, he wanted to leave instantly, didn't want to talk to anyone, didn't want to look me in the face. He had been diagnosed since 2010. I've met Black African people who said they would never want a Black HIV clinician to deal with them because eventually they might know them, and sometimes you get people saying I don't want to go to a service provided by white people. It's both sides, really, the challenges are there.

Concerns about how members within a particular community might react to HIV, as in the example given above, can be intensified when religion – not known for its acceptance of HIV – is added to the mix, as highlighted by a church-going Black African woman:

> People in my church don't know about my HIV, I've been going there all of the 17 years, and one of the preachers talked about the disease that you could catch and pass on, and I kept my mouth shut, I learnt to zip it … I haven't spoken to others in the church, because people are funny. When they know, they change, a lot of them are ignorant, but if you give them the information and then they use it against you, you only have yourself to blame.

Some clinicians worried whether the understandable protection given to PLWH in the earlier days of the epidemic by providing care in dedicated HIV units, excluding other medical and nursing teams for fear of discrimination, had also resulted in a lack of training and broadening of understanding of the significance of HIV among other professionals, thus, in some ways, delaying the inevitable process of developing a wider acceptance of HIV in healthcare, a point made by a senior nurse:

> We've made masses and masses of advances in treatment, but I think we made little headway from a stigma point of view. I think that is partly a by-product of the model we have created, that we may have hidden HIV away for too long, and therefore other healthcare professions outside the specialty have not had the same opportunity to develop skill. I think HIV has become much more invisible now, and people have misconceptions around it, for example around the fact that people still die of HIV … and in the case of health professions they either think somebody is going to die, or they think HIV is over, and so actually there is a big knowledge gap.

Care from statutory services

Changes to the relationship between PLWH and the medical and nursing teams

As in the years immediately following the introduction of ART, relationships between PLWH and clinical teams continued to change through to 2020. What is most striking now is that different cohorts of PLWH can have very different needs and expectations. Younger people recently diagnosed and who have had access to effective treatments from the start, do not carry the emotional, health, and practical baggage of the traumatic experiences of those who experienced the early days of the epidemic. Clearly, the converse can apply to those who have been living with HIV for many years, as one doctor illustrated:

> *I have two different HIV clinics in different parts of London. One is a much younger cohort, and the patient feedback is that they feel well cared for. I don't think there is that individual deep understanding of the patient in the way it used to be when the numbers were smaller. Whereas when I go to my other clinic where PLWH have been positive for 20 or 30 years, I think people still have that legacy type of care where we really know them, and I remember when their partner died and they were on the ward when I was on the ward and so on. You see those people who have lost friends, jobs, don't have pensions, have been horribly scarred by earlier drugs and opportunistic infections. And then you see people for whom it's just something they come in [for] and pick up their pills every six months and carry on with the rest of their lives, and that's very different.*

People who have lived with HIV for many years are aware of the changes in their relationship with the clinicians caring for them. For some, these changes are experienced as a return to old-fashioned medical attitudes and behaviours that were challenged in earlier years of the epidemic, as reported by a gay man living with HIV:

> *These days, empowerment of patients outside the mothership, as I call the HIV clinic, is crap, it's old school, it's patronising, it's inefficient. When I had to go and get my heart fixed it was a trip and a half into this patronising world.*

For others, it is the sometimes mechanical, almost impersonal interaction between the newly diagnosed patient and doctor that brings a sense of regret to the exchange, as stated by another gay man:

> *People that are diagnosed today, it's very much going back to a patient/doctor relationship where they go, I've got HIV, OK, take these, off you go, bang. But in those days, because there were so many other things, because there was so much stigma, because there weren't any drugs, because they were trying desperately, the model of medicine that was used, the only way it was going to work for those with HIV was a partnership model.*

The views of these patients were echoed by the regrets expressed by a senior HIV physician who had spent most of his professional life caring for PLWH. Here, part of the blame is placed on the managerial decisions made in recent years, making reference to policy changes rather than to HIV treatment:

> *It is a big shame that having spent 25 years building up this fantastic care where the patient is central, now it is totally disintegrated, I think due to poor management, and doctors and patients being unwilling to stand up and say, this is wrong. In the early days, PLWH would choose the doctor they wanted to see because of their style of care, different people wanted different approaches, there is no right way to practise medicine, and I think the lack of individuality is actually having an impact on the level and degree of care.*

Efforts to maintain a link between PLWH and the clinical teams have continued but have experienced change. Frequently, they aimed at maintaining informal and practical contacts, through patients working as peer support workers. The process of developing these new roles has required considerable work to overcome barriers, however, as a senior HIV nurse explained:

> *We introduced peer support and tried to make it acceptable to nurses and health advisors. Peer support workers can encroach on other people's roles, so a peer support patient coming in and seeing a patient about being newly diagnosed can potentially encroach on the role of the nurse or health advisor, but it has been accepted.*

Alternative models of care aimed at facilitating patient engagement, available in some large HIV clinics, include that of the paid patient representative, a modification of the patient as peer support worker mode. A physician working in one such service explained:

> *We now have three paid patient representatives in our clinic, and they see over 1000 clients a year, they are essentially part of the service provision, they are very good at signposting, running workshops, newly diagnosed courses, forums, hepatitis C workshops, women's lunch club, and a choir.*

The case of mental health care

From the early days of the epidemic, mental health workers (clinical psychologists, psychiatrists, and psychiatric nurses) had a strong presence within the HIV specialist teams. Over the years, HIV clinics struggled to maintain access to this specialist mental health assessment and care, with varying success. HIV clinics without mental health workers attached to the specialist service would have to rely on the general local psychiatric services, which were often overstretched and struggling to cope with major psychiatric disorders.

Nevertheless, large HIV clinics have managed to retain some mental health services, often by funding it directly, or in collaboration with the local mental health trust, as reported by a physician working in one such clinic:

> *We have kept our mental health services pretty intact, so we have an inhouse psychiatrist, four psychologists, and three health advisors, and they are highly effective, although the psychiatry side is a bit restricted, as at some point we have to hand the patients back to the GP and the local psychiatric services, which can be problematic.*

Smaller, less affluent clinics have struggled to maintain a basic service, relying on the existing psychiatric community services, which are also stretched, and only able to deal with the more severe problems. Here is a contrasting view, described by a physician working in a less privileged setting:

> *We have lost our designated psychiatrist, and we now have somebody who will not take new patients, will only see old ones. Mental health care is fragmented, and the pressure on mental health services, like community mental health services is huge, the patients practically have to stab someone in the street to be seen by a community mental health team (CMHT), otherwise you are not considered to be an important priority.*

Government austerity directives have meant that some common, significant, but easy to manage HIV-related problems, such as sexual dysfunction and HIV-related fatigue, have become difficult to provide treatment for. In earlier times, collaboration between the HIV clinicians and the mental health team allowed prompt assessment, psychological interventions, and provision of medication for these conditions. However, in the last few years access to such drugs and to therapy has become more restricted, with neither the mental health services nor the HIV managers being prepared to fund the medication. A psychiatrist dealing with such problems explained the constraints faced:

> *Erectile dysfunction in particular responds to medication such as sildenafil (Viagra), although it has potential interaction with some ART drugs, and we developed a collaborative approach with the HIV physicians. However, in the last few years and as a result of financial pressures, prescribing was restricted by the hospital pharmacy, and patients had to rely on private prescriptions or buy the medication online. Similarly, HIV-associated fatigue was another problem we saw in our mental health clinics, after the HIV teams had ruled out any obvious physical factors. Psychostimulants, like methylphenidate and modafinil were very effective. Unfortunately, as financial austerity continued to affect the NHS, both the mental health and HIV pharmacies stopped dispensing them.*

HIV care – specialist services or general practice care?

As highlighted in reports discussing the care of PLWH (NAT 2016; Baylis et al. 2017), the main drivers for change in service provision have been the development of the concept of HIV as a long-term condition, and the consequences of the implementation of the Health and Social Care Act 2012.

Viewing HIV as a long-term condition, as opposed to one requiring acute intervention, suggests that diagnosis and management of co-morbidities, access to appropriate treatment, and support to reduce the risk of complications, is all that is required. It is argued that such care could be provided by infrequent monitoring appointments with the specialist clinicians. However, for many PLWH this model downplays their day-to-day difficulties, minimising the wider consequences of their condition, and shifts care from the HIV specialist centres to overworked and less experienced GPs, who are not always well placed to recognise associated co-morbidities or treatment side-effects. Most PLWH who have experienced specialist clinic-based care over the decades, are reluctant to accept the idea that devolving their care to GPs is the best option. They raise concerns about the limited HIV expertise of family doctors, in contrast with the expertise of the teams working in HIV clinics, continuing with greater urgency earlier debates in relation to non-HIV conditions about the relative roles of specialist clinics and general practice. Two gay men living with HIV outlined their views on the likely changes:

> *I think it would be a mistake if HIV was treated as just another chronic illness to be managed by the GP, and only go to the HIV centre if there is a problem. The assump-tion that all GPs are going to know about it and deal with it, and are trained for it, it's just not the case. Specialist services have served us very well.*

> *There has been a lot of discussion over the years about 'specialism' versus 'generalism', and about trying to move HIV care out of the specialist centres, and from my point of view, I still think that the excellence of the care is related to specialism, and that is where I want to be.*

The reluctance of long-term patients to transfer all their HIV care to their GPs is made explicit by some using dismissive language. In particular, there are concerns about the back and forth referral from GP to clinic, and the weakening of the spe-cialist service. A Black African woman made her views clear:

> *Now you are advised to go to your GP, which is a problem. The GPs are useless, they have too many patients, they don't know what to do with you, so they usually send you back to your consultant, and it's back and forth, and I think it's worse in the sense that the HIV clinics no longer give a comprehensive service where they can deal with all your difficulties.*

One counterargument, however, is that HIV care has been overfunded, and that both patients and their carers have been indulged by past care. However, a gay man living with HIV batted that argument back, pleading for such care to be extended to other conditions:

> *We get accused of exceptionalism, and of course the argument against HIV exceptional-ism is that everybody should be treated exceptionally, and the only reason we defeated*

> *HIV is because we treated it exceptionally. It was a cultural and historical event of the first importance.*

Concerns about the loss of confidentiality in the setting of general practice, and also about the potential for greater stigma, particularly in the case of people from ethnic minority backgrounds, were raised by a worker supporting Black African PLWH:

> *Running service user groups for Black African PLWH, I hear lots of complaints about GP services. Many patients say they experience a lot of stigma around that. In the last three to four years, since the NHS has been able to force people to go back to their GPs, complaints have increased. I've come across people who have completely stopped going to their GPs. Last year someone told me about being addressed in the reception area as the person with HIV.*

For PLWH with additional health and social problems, it is the complicated arrangements to get prescriptions for other conditions or be referred to a specialist, that adds to the burden of coping with their health difficulties through GP services. A gay man described some of these complicated arrangements:

> *I had my psychological therapy through the HIV clinic. It is only recently that referrals have had to be through your GP. Also, all my heart medications used to be prescribed by the clinic, together with my HIV medicines, but now I have to go to the GP, have a blood test, and unless there is anything wrong, they just repeat the prescription. So, in a way that's complicated our lives. It's the fracturing of the medical service.*

In contrast with the generally negative views of those having lived with HIV for many years about the involvement of GPs, some HIV physicians presented a more nuanced position on the interface between family doctors and HIV specialists, and between the old and new cohorts of PLWH. It is the old cohorts of PLWH that are aware of the changes in care. Newly diagnosed, generally younger patients, who have not known anything different, do not know about, or feel strongly about the changes:

> *For those who didn't experience the model of care that we provided in the early days, which was incredible, and moving, and superlative, they don't know what they have lost. They are just young guys who are well, they get their treatment and [HIV] is a chronic condition, they can't pass it on, they just get on with it. But for those that experienced that, it's almost a bereavement because they have lost their sense of the special thing, and it's become a commodity. The message for patients, medically speaking, is this is a chronic condition and that's why everything is being taken away. For NHS England, it's a small chronic condition which is not generally terminal and can be well controlled. On every level we are reducing the specialness, sorry, we can no longer fund the dietician every week, now they come once a month. We can't prescribe you non-HIV medications, we shall write to your GP, if you don't want us to write to your GP, we cannot manage your co-morbidities, that's how life is.*

One potential advantage of the new 'normalisation of care' approach (i.e. treating HIV like other long-term conditions with the involvement of GPs and specialists other than HIV clinicians), could be a reduction in the stigma and isolation of patients. Additionally, the involvement of other professionals becomes more relevant when dealing with ageing patients with multiple co-morbidities, when the skills of the HIV clinicians may not be sufficient to provide adequately for the care of such complex problems, as argued by an HIV physician:

> *The patient-centred approach was important, this [is] not-quite cradle to grave, but from diagnosis to death, and that everything that the patient needed, we would deal with. I think that was the right response at that point in time. I do not think it's the right model now, in terms of chronic medical conditions, and I think one of the problems that [the] patient-centred model created was that it siloed HIV services, it made them too special. It was right at the beginning, in order to create specialisms to ensure patients and vulnerable groups were treated in an appropriate way, but now it can allow stigma to persist, it allows ignorance to persist, it allows incompetence to persist.*

However, if care for HIV is to be moved from the HIV specialist to the GP, how is it to be best achieved? One physician pointed out that, in fact, HIV may in some cases continue to be too complex for primary care, and so partnerships would not cease to be important with specialist HIV care:

> *I think the care of PLWH is quite highly specialised in terms of therapies, side-effects and monitoring, and I think it may be possible to develop good co-partnerships with general practice but I don't think it's quite like other diseases, like diabetes for example.*

These new partnerships might, for example, include the employment of nurses with enhanced skills and responsibilities, as was the opinion of one physician:

> *We can't just keep bouncing between one paradigm – we do it all, and the other paradigm – the GPs do it all. Maybe what we need is a third way with clinical nurse specialists and collaborative care and one care record. And so maybe eventually the next wave of change might enable us to get that.*

One model already introduced in some areas for some PLWH with ongoing difficulties is one where HIV community nurses perform that link role, and one that could be extended to other HIV groups. A community nurse described her experience in that role:

> *We now have a cohort of people who don't or can't go to hospital. We meet with the HIV consultant once a month, go through our own template and do all the actions and issues to discuss with the consultant, do a full medication review, get blood results, and then see the patients at home weekly, or as needed. The consultant decides on the medication regime, and then we do the repeat prescriptions. Once a year the consultant will come with us and see the patient at home. We have patients that haven't been to hospital for three years and who are undetectable and well.*

Fragmented commissioning and care

The Health and Social Care Act 2012 introduced changes to the NHS in England which have resulted in increased fragmentation. The principal change was the separation of treatment and care from prevention, with added changes to the commissioning of services.

Specialist HIV treatment and care are directly commissioned by NHS England through a National Commissioning Board, while most local services are commissioned locally by Clinical Commissioning Groups (CCG). Primary care for HIV is also commissioned centrally but is moving to the CCGs.

Prevention for HIV, together with other sexual health services, like contraception, sexually transmitted infections testing and treatment, and sexual health promotion, are now the responsibility of Public Health Commissioners, themselves under the responsibility of the local authorities.

The picture is clearly complicated. The fragmentation of responsibilities for commissioning and funding has been criticised by many workers in the field, particularly as it has led to closure of specialist services (NAT 2016; White 2017; Baylis et al., 2017). Public Health England (2017b) also raised concerns about fragmentation of commissioning. Among our participants, a charity worker, an HIV physician, and an HIV administrator, shared their negative views of the impact of the 2012 Act:

> *I think that, inadvertently, the Lansley reforms of 2012 have been a disaster for AIDS and sexual health services by splitting them apart, putting HIV prevention into public health is terribly, terribly wasteful and destructive of good teams. But that wasn't done maliciously, it was done incompetently.*

> *Commissioning for HIV had been pretty good, and ending of the ring-fencing of HIV services didn't really lead to underfunding. But the real problem has been with the devolution of public health to the local authorities, and I think that has made quite an impact on the provision of generic sexual health services and those services that are part of HIV will suffer.*

> *The disorganisation of services caused by the 2012 Health and Social Care Act, the Lansley Act, was a disaster in general but a particular disaster for HIV. It is disastrous because of the split it causes between the public health side of STIs and the HIV specialist care, and the disruption that's caused to services is just huge.*

A clear example of the conflicts that arose from the fragmented commissioning out of the 2012 Act is illustrated by the choices HIV community nurses working on the front line are forced to make daily:

> *We are a community nursing service that manages already diagnosed people, but we do have a small testing arm, and sometimes we'll do tests for partners or family members at home. It's nothing on the scale of a sexual health clinic, though. It was always within our contract to deliver HIV testing, but when the commissioning changed, the money for prevention, that is for testing, didn't come with the contract. So, we still do it, but we don't get paid.*

There is concern that the Health and Social Care Act 2012 points the health service in directions that may damage the chances of maintaining the kind of service that has provided excellent HIV care to anyone requiring it. Separating the commissioning of prevention and care has made the previously seamless model of care less coordinated, and opened up the potential to privatise profitable services. While the advantages of the integrated model would be applicable to other medical conditions, according to this physician:

> *I think one of the real challenges at the moment is the general direction of the NHS in terms of the Health Social Care Act, separating HIV and sexual health GUM services, and the privatisation of services where integrated care is not a priority of the private provider. We have been lucky that patients can still have open access to services. Can you think where else in the NHS can patients access secondary care services without going through a GP, other than into A&E? Some people would argue that that's a model that should be replicated in other areas, rather than having general practice do all that. And I still feel that HIV will still continue to have open access services, and I think open access services have driven up standards.*

In spite of the impact of the reorganisation of HIV services, financial austerity, and legislative changes, for some there are still enough ingredients left in the system to ensure that things will continue to work well enough for those with HIV, as claimed by a gay man living with HIV:

> *I think it is remarkable that the situation hasn't got worse, and I think that is because, right at the centre, there is still a very dedicated group, a very good HIV service in this country, we have a centralised STI clinic system, that's why we were able to do what we have done. I don't know what it would be like if I had another long-term condition like diabetes, but I think when you have a serious condition, the NHS still works.*

HIV charities

HIV charities have continued to provide a very important service, but like the NHS, their role and scope have changed in the last decade, with reduced funding, an acceleration of the merger of organisations, and a rethinking of their remits being important drivers. As in the earlier days of the HIV epidemic, charities have filled many of the gaps left untouched by the statutory services. The new urgency is that PLWH are likely to have less contact with statutory medical and social services, partly due to changes in their clinical needs, but also because of service reduction. A physician commented on this shift:

> *A range of charities and support groups are providing some of the functions that perhaps social workers would have provided. I think there is a focus from the peer support organisations around new patient groups, addressing stigma, which has been helpfully addressed though the U=U issue. There is the increased function of these organisations*

in trying to deliver help and advice around social issues, as services have been removed in terms of social care.

Charities have had to adapt to the funding landscape and to the stricter demands of the funders, focusing on evaluation and employing fund-raisers to survive. One charity worker explained:

Funders are better at giving longer-term funding now, better to recognise that if the services you are delivering are working, why change them? It has been helpful to think about outcomes-based work, because it has made us think about why are we doing this, what difference does it make to people, and how do we know it's making a difference? We have a fund-raising team who has always been good at community-based funding … but the last couple of years have been tough.

The focus of the HIV charities has had to change in response to changing HIV epidemiological profiles. For example, a Scottish charity has developed links with general practice to help them deal with new issues raised by HIV:

We have funding to work with GPs, to train around increasing discussion about HIV testing with African patients, and addressing some of the concerns that GPs might have, like feeling that they might come across as racist, and how to have those difficult conversations … we have also developed training for GP practices around working with MSM, and delivering in GP practices alongside NHS staff.

The specific needs of people ageing with HIV have become the focus of some charities, where imaginative responses have been developed. Instead of regarding older PLWH as in need of passive support and 'hand-holding', this charity worker describes the results of initiatives taken by PLWH themselves organising activities to avoid social isolation:

We started with a focus group, and at first older people with HIV were fixated on a drop-in when there weren't younger people around, so I was more interested in what they wanted the drop-in for, and then it became clear it was about being isolated, about wanting to mix with people like you … So, they started a social group about nine years ago that goes out and does things every week and goes to all sort of places that we can get free tickets for or cheap things.

Users of HIV charities can be fulsome in their appreciation of the services provided. A Black African woman with HIV gave examples of the kind of help she was now receiving:

I think it is one of the best charities out there in that it's quite mixed. For example, they have a gay men's lunch, and an African women's lunch, and a mixed, neither gay nor

African women over 50s, whoever wants to come, and there was a Children and Families Group, which is what I was working with until the funding ran out. They help you apply for small grants, they helped me get a computer and helped me apply to get a fridge, they even help people who don't have recourse to public funds to get clothes and baby things.

HIV prevention: progress and obstacles

Antenatal screening for HIV was widespread by the late '90s, and it allowed the early identification of HIV infection in pregnant women. Prevention of transmission from mother to the unborn child was a major success story in the UK, with a steep fall in transmission rates which continued well into the new century. Transmission rates fell from 25.6% in 1993 (Duong et al. 1999) to less than 0.5% by 2014 (Peters et al. 2017).

Inadequacies in school education about sexual and emotional relationships, as well as prevention of sexually transmitted diseases including HIV are often attributed to political rulings (Sex Education Forum, 2018). Despite this and the newer relaxation and lack of urgency surrounding HIV, with it now no longer making newspaper headlines, new preventive issues have arisen. These include the availability of new biomedical approaches to prevention, and the changing use of recreational drugs and other substances. Sadly, however, early optimism about vaccines following the RV144 trial in Thailand that showed a good response, a large trial in South Africa (HVTN 702) including 5,407 participants, showed no benefit compared with placebo, and the trial was stopped early in 2020. Further trials are being planned to start in late 2020.

Important steps in the biomedical prevention of HIV infection have been the introduction of PEP (post-exposure prophylaxis) and PrEP (pre-exposure prophylaxis), both shown to be both clinically valuable and cost effective (Grant et al. 2010; McCormack et al. 2016; Siedner et al. 2018).

PEP has been used both in the prevention of HIV infection by occupational exposure of health care workers and after unprotected anal and vaginal sex, effective when administration of ART occurs within 72 hours of the risky incident (Cresswell et al. 2016; Cardo et al. 1997; EAGA 2008; Panlilio et al. 2005; Public Health England 2014). However, providing immediate access to PEP is not enough, as people fail to request it when they do not recognise their exposure as high risk (Celum et al. 2001). Others have been blocked from accessing PEP, as a charity worker living with HIV explained:

One of our clients tried to get PEP … and the receptionist repeatedly put the phone down on him and said, "serves you fucking well right".

For individuals presenting with repeated requests for PEP as a result of sexual exposure, risk reduction counselling (Reitmeijer 2007), including motivational interviewing, an approach often used in counselling people with substance misuse problems (Miller and Rollnick 2013; Llewellyn et al. 2019), is recommended in addition to medication. However, this approach has met with limited success, neither preventing further requests for PEP, nor the number of subsequent sexually transmitted infections (Llewellyn et al. 2019).

As regards PrEP, Public Health England made positive PrEP usage recommendations for the elimination of HIV transmission in the UK, as well as early diagnosis and treatment (BHIVA/BASHH 2018; Public Health England 2018). However, at first, there was a degree of hesitation and misinformation provided by NHS England about the new intervention. An HIV physician criticised the early official response, which appeared tabloid in approach:

> *Unfortunately, NHS England dealt with the reasonable request for funding for PrEP, on the grounds that [it] is highly cost effective and probably cost saving, in a very emotional way, saying that funding PrEP would prevent children with cystic fibrosis from breathing properly.*

Pressure was applied to NHS England, the agency responsible for care, and to Public Health England, the agency responsible for prevention, by activists and charities to ensure that access to PrEP became more widely available on the NHS. Practical concerns about its use remain, in particular whether people would commit to taking the medication correctly. One of the most common risk factors for not adhering to the PrEP medication regimen is the use of alcohol or recreational drugs. Alcohol consumption has been linked to missing PrEP pills (Storholm et al. 2017), and it has been found that alcohol and cocaine have an additive effect on non-adherence (Goodman-Meza et al. 2019). In the words of a gay activist living with HIV:

> *There ought to be targeted education [and] PrEP for people who are completely smashed day and night. I'm also aware that these people are least likely to be consistent in their use of PrEP … Adherence is the key issue here and if your life is so scattered by drugs then your adherence is likely to be undermined … there is a vicious circle here.*

As PLWH started to enjoy better health and quality of life, one particular area of behaviour had implications for mental and physical health. Recreational drugs to enhance sexual enjoyment, such as crystal meth, increasingly appeared on the gay scene in the UK in recent years. Chemsex became the term to refer to the use of particular drugs, such as mephedrone, gamma-hydroxybutyrate (GHB), butyrolactone (GBL), and methamphetamine to heighten sexual pleasure. A psychiatric nurse describes the situation she faced in her clinic, and how the traditional drug services had to adapt to PLWH:

> *In the last few years, recreational drugs became a real problem, especially crystal meth. I got involved in setting up a drug clinic in the general hospital, because drugs had a massive impact on the physical and mental health of PLWH. We worked with the local drug service, which had historically been for heroin and methadone, and it branched out into dealing with recreational drugs, and it really changed the way they worked. HIV patients wouldn't go to their local drug services, but were prepared to come to the drug service at the hospital where they received their HIV care.*

HIV is not be now the killer that it was, but for some PLWH a new ingredient – that can reintroduce lethality – is recreational drug use, as a number of our participants pointed out. An HIV male nurse expressed concern as to where the drug-use epidemic was heading:

> *The big thing now is chemsex. Now we are seeing people die of drugs, which is really hard for me to see. We've had four deaths from G this year, and there is a part of me that just wants to weep, I can't see another group of young men die.*

Clearly, not every person attending sexual health clinics requesting PEP following sexual exposure had been using chemsex, however, many PLWH report some chemsex use. Their wish to reduce or give up its use, nevertheless, has not always been a priority, as described by a recreational drugs worker:

> *In 2010 we started prescribing PEP (Post-Exposure Prophylaxis), and the assessment proforma about drug use had only two questions: are you an injecting drug user? Have you had sex with an HIV drug user? So, I asked the nurses to add a third question: Do you use party drugs for sex? What's your favourite one? Are you having a good time? And we found that 100% of people who came asking for PEP, had come from a chemsex environment, whether it was one on one, whether it was a sniff of drugs in a sauna, or a three-day bender with multiple people. But they are not walking in with their hand up saying, help me stop chemsex, please, they are saying, treat the consequences of my chemsex, please.*

The newer psychoactive substances, previously known as legal highs – an always changing group of substances – and chemsex, have also found their way into the populations that had injected opiates (Ralphs and Grey 2018), forcing health workers to learn and adapt to the evolving substances, as well as continuing to manage the old ones. A psychiatrist working with IDU, talked about her experience:

> *We now see people using the new legal highs, chemsex, in particular new patients, and they don't see themselves as belonging to the substance misuse side, so we have had to educate ourselves to meet their needs, as there are no good places we could send them to, so we have taken more of that work ourselves, as well as monitoring the methadone prescribing in the HIV unit for the long-term injecting drug users.*

There is, nevertheless, limited expertise in the HIV and sexual health services regarding the needs of MSM who use recreational drugs. Thus, there is little understanding of – and support for – those using chemsex, as an MSM living with HIV argued:

> *One thing I find quite extraordinary is a reluctance of people working with HIV prevention up till quite recently … and for gay men generally, just to talk about why gay men use many drugs so intensively and for so long? And why it is acceptable, that's the cultural norm.*

The problem of HIV infection in people who inject drugs has received attention again, with the ongoing outbreak of HIV among people who inject drugs
in Glasgow, where more than 100 cases of HIV infection in this group have
been identified recently. The closure of the busiest needle and syringe exchange
service in Glasgow's Central Station, reducing access to clean injecting equipment and its disposal has been a contributory factor. The refusal of the
Westminster government to create a Drug Consumption Room (DCR) in
Glasgow, a clinic where addicts could bring their own drugs to inject with clean
needles under supervision, with the added offer of health checks, is also thought
to have contributed to the outbreak of new cases (NAT 2018; Public Health
England 2016).

Consistent with the kind of problems identified in Glasgow, health workers
highlight the difficulties encountered in caring for IDU with HIV, as well
as the mixed success that can be achieved, as an experienced HIV physician
described:

> *As regards drug services, we are going through a bit of a crisis now in Scotland … drug
> related deaths are going up, we have HIV, we have A&E attendances going up, we have
> more injecting, we have a huge epidemic of injecting with new psychoactive substances
> (NPS). And all of a sudden, the government is beginning to listen to us again, and to
> ask about harm reduction. We now have a safe injecting room, which we have manged
> to get going, and other things like prescribing and treatment service, but we have prob-
> lems in prisons, where we are banging our heads against the wall, and general practice,
> where the new contract coming out next year doesn't include drug users as a core service,
> and drug treatment services are being cut back.*

Towards eradication of HIV

ART has now led to significant improvement in the health of the majority of
PLWH with access to treatment, although co-morbidities and social and financial
difficulties continue to add complexities to what is now regarded as a chronic
manageable disease. However, PLWH are still the victims of stigma. Care from
statutory services and charities has undergone important changes, and there is an
ongoing discussion about the relationship between specialist HIV services and
general practice, and its impact on person-centred care. Furthermore, the Health
and Social Care Act 2012 has brought about changes to the provision of NHS
HIV care and prevention in England, resulting in fragmentation of service provision. Prevention still remains an important subject of discussion. Pharmacological
developments, such as PrEP, offer the possibility of a major reduction in the incidence of new cases of HIV infection, and the collaboration of activists and
healthcare workers has led to the formation of new alliances to push for change.
The apparently increasing role of chemsex for MSM, and the reduction in the
provision of harm reduction interventions for drug users, remain key areas of
concern.

References

Bangalore S, Kamalakkannan G, Parkar S, and Masserli F (2007) Fixed-dose combinations improve medication compliance: a meta-analysis. *The American Journal of Medicine*, 120(8), 713–719.

Cresswell, F., Waters, L., Briggs, E., Fox, J., Harbottle, J., Hawkins, D., Murchie, M., Radcliffe, K., Rafferty, P., Rodger, A. and Fisher, M. (2016) UK Guideline for the use of HIV post-exposure prophylaxis following sexual exposure, 2015. *International Journal of STD and AIDS*, 27(9), 713–738.

Baylis A, Buck D, Anderson J, Jabbal J and Ross S (2017) *The future of HIV services in England*. London, The King's Fund.

BHIVA (2003) *Guidelines for the treatment of HIV-infected adults with ART*. London, Mediscript Ltd.

BHIVA/BASHH (2018) *Guidelines on the use of HIV pre-exposure prophylaxis (PrEP)*. London, Mediscript Ltd.

Bilsen, W van (2019) *HIV as a chronic condition: a study of the experiences of HIV-related burden among recently diagnosed MSM living in The Netherlands*. AIDS IMPACT XIV International Conference, London, July 29–31.

Cardo DM, Culver DH, Ciesielski CA, Srivastava PU, Marcus R, and McKibben PS (1997) A case–control study of HIV seroconversion in health care workers after percutaneous exposure. *New England Journal of Medicine*, 337(21), 1485–1490.

Celum CL, Buchbinder SP, Donnell D, Douglas Jr. JM and Flores J (2001) Early HIV infection in the HIV Network for the Prevention Trials Vaccine Preparedness Cohort: risk behaviors, symptoms, and early plasma and genital tract virus load. *The Journal of Infectious Diseases*, 183(1), 23–35.

Duong T, Ades A, Gibb DM, Tookey PA and Masters J (1999) Vertical transmission rates for HIV in the British Isles: estimates based on surveillance data. *British Medical Journal*, 319(7219), 1227–1229.

EAGA (2008) HIV post-exposure prophylaxis: guidance from the UK Chief Medical Officer's. *Expert Advisory Group on AIDS*. London, Department of Health and Social Care.

Goodman-Meza D, Beymar MR, Kofron RM, and Rooney JF (2019) Effective use of PrEP among stimulant users with multiple condomless sexual partners: a longitudinal study of MSM in Los Angeles. *AIDS Care*, 31(10), 1228–1233.

Grant RM, Lama JR, Anderson PL and iPrEx Study Team (2010) Pre-exposure chemoprophylaxis for HIV prevention in men that have sex with men. *New England Journal of Medicine*, 363(27): 2587–2599.

HIV Psychosocial network (2018) An 'austerity audit' of services and living conditions for people living with HIV in the UK, a decade after the financial crisis. http://hivpsychosocialnetworkuk.tumblr.com

Llewellyn CD, Abraham C, Pollard A, Jones CI and Smith H (2019) A randomised controlled trial of a telephone administered brief HIV risk reduction intervention amongst MSM prescribed PEP for HIV after sexual exposure in the UK: Project PEPSE. *PLoS one*, 14(5), e0216855.

McCormack S, Dunn D, Desai M, Dolling D, Gafos M, Gilson R, Sullivan A, Clarke A, Reeves I (2016) Pre-exposure prophylaxis to prevent acquisition of HIV-1 infection (PROUD): effectiveness results from the pilot phase of a pragmatic open- label randomised trial. *The Lancet*, 387, 53–60 https://doi.org/10.1016/S0140-6736(15)00056-2

Miller W and Rollnick S (2013) *Motivational Interviewing: helping people change*. New York, Guilford Press.

NAM (2017) Undetectable equals Untransmittable (U=U) Consensus Statement. www.preventionaccess.org/consensus

NAT (2016) HIV in the future NHS: what next for people living with HIV in England. www.nat.org.uk/publications

NAT (2018) *Policy Briefing: HIV outbreak in Glasgow – more needs to be done.* London, National AIDS Trust.

Panlilio AL, Cardo DM, Grohnskopf LA, Heneine W and Ross CS (2005) Updated US Public Health Service Guidelines for the management of occupational exposures to HIV, and recommendations for PEP. *Morbidity and Mortality Weekly Report: Recommendations and Reports*, 54(9), 1-CE-4.

Peters H, Francis K, Sconza R, Horn A, Peckham C, Tookey PA, and Thorne C (2017) UK Mother to Child HIV transmission Rates Continue to Decline: 2012–2014. *Clinical Infectious Diseases*, 64(4), 527–528.

Public Health England (2014) *Making it work. A guide to whole system commissioning for sexual health, reproductive health, and HIV.* London, PHE Publications.

Public Health England (2016) *Shooting up: infections among people who inject drugs in the UK.* London, PHE Publications.

Public Health England (2017a) *Sexual Health, Reproductive Health, and HIV.* London, PHE Publications.

Public Health England (2017b) *Towards elimination of HIV transmission, AIDS, and HIV-related deaths in the UK.* London. PHE Publications.

Public Health England (2018) Trends in new HIV diagnoses and people receiving HIV-related care in the UK: data to the end of December 2017. *Heath Protection Report*, 12, 32.

Ralphs R and Grey P (2018) New psychoactive substances: new service provider challenges. *Drugs: Education, Prevention, and Policy*, 25(4), 301–312.

Reitmeijer CA (2007) Risk reduction counselling for prevention of sexually transmitted infections: how it works and how to make it work. *Sexually Transmitted Infections*, 83(1), 2–9.

Sex Education Forum (2018) *Young people's relationships and sex education (RSE) poll 2018.* http://www.sexeducationforum.org.uk/youngpeoplespoll2018

Siedner M, Tumarkin E and Bogoch U (2018) HIV post-exposure prophylaxis (PEP). *British Medical Journal*, 363:k4928 http://dx.dol.org/10.1136/bmj.k4928

Squire C (2013) *Living with HIV and ARVs.* Basingstoke, Palgrave Macmillan.

Storholm ED, Volk JE, Marcus JL, Silverberg MJ and Satre DD (2017) Risk perception, sexual behaviors, and PrEP adherence among substance-using MSM: a qualitative study. *Prevention Science*, 18(6), 737–747.

UNAIDS (2018) Undetectable=Untransmittable. Public Health and HIV viral load suppression. Unaids.org.

Vernazza P, Hirschel B, Bernasconi E, and Flepp M (2008) Les personnes seropositives ne souffrant d'aucune autre MST et suivant un traitement antiretroviral efficace ne transmettent pas le VIH par voie sexuelle. *Bulletin des Medicines Suisses*, 89(5) 165–169.

White, C (2017) Sexual health services on the brink. *British Medical Journal*, 359:5395 https://doi.org/10.1136/bmj.j5395

Part II

The legacy of HIV and lessons learnt

6 The development of person-centred HIV care

What is meant by person-centred care?

Person-centred care is now commonplace terminology in health care, and at least lip service is paid to the approach on the clinical frontline, at both management and policy level. This was not always so. Less appreciated is the key role HIV played in developing ideas and practices around what person-centred care could mean, well beyond early calls that people living with HIV (PLWH) should have a significant say in their care. In the UK, the history of HIV care illustrates clearly a person-centred lineage from the start of the epidemic in the early 1980s, and its evolution over time, as changes in the clinical prognosis of HIV and its wider social perception changed.

Person-centred care is now defined in very specific terms. In the NHS England declaration of commitment to person-centred care (NHS England 2015), the definition by National Voices is advanced as: "I can plan my care with people who work together to understand me and my carer(s), allow me control, and bring together services to achieve the outcomes important to me" (NAT 2016). The declaration on 'Whole person care' in HIV care and support backed by UK charities and clinicians' organisations, includes not only the medical perspective of care, but recognises the social, economic, employment, and physical and mental health needs associated with HIV. Several principles are incorporated, such as care planning; parity of esteem – to ensure that healthcare workers recognise their needs and HIV does not become an 'invisible' condition; addressing care inequality; and patient self-management (NAT 2017). For the British HIV Association (BHIVA), person-centred care means that "services consciously adopt the perspectives of individuals, families and communities to respond to their needs and preferences in humane and holistic ways; the person is a participant, not just a beneficiary of the health system" (BHIVA 2018).

As identified in the above definitions, in the narrowest sense, person-centred care starts with the interaction between the person and immediate professional carers, like doctors, nurses, and others, and moves forward more widely to include other teams and services, sometimes in the form of the 'one-stop shop', in which the patient occupies a central place to which these services come, rather than the patient being sent to a variety of clinics and services in the hospital, outside the central specialist clinic.

The person-centred care approach contrasts with the traditional medical model, in which doctors (usually male) knew best, and told the patient what was wrong, and what treatment was required, while the nurses (usually female), and other professionals remained in attendance (Balint 1969). This approach was starting to be challenged by the time HIV came along, although it was still firmly entrenched. The Ottawa Charter for Health Promotion (1986) under the auspices of the World Health Organisation, represents part of the move away from traditional models of medicine, including both the personal and socio-ecological approach to health. Important components of the person-centred model include a biopsychosocial perspective, regarding the patient as a person, and the sharing of decision-making, power, and responsibility, amongst others (Bower and Mead 2007). Holistic nursing models of care were developed in the UK in the 1980s (Roper et al. 2000), providing inspiration to nurses in HIV. Since the early days of the concept, the patient-centred model has moved from "the periphery of medicine to the epicentre of clinical practice and medical education", including four main components: exploring the illness experience; understanding the whole person; finding common ground; and enhancing the patient–clinician relationship (Stewart et al. 2014).

HIV care has illustrated clearly the value of this approach, and there is empirical evidence to confirm a desire to share decision-making between PLWH and their professional carers. Using the instrument developed by Ende et al. (1989) to measure desire for autonomy in clinical situations, which comprised two dimensions, i.e. wish for involvement in decision-making, and information-seeking, Catalan et al. (1994) and Carretero et al. (1998) were able to show not only high levels of desire for patients' involvement amongst PLWH and their carers, but also important variations in terms of desire for decision-making and information-seeking. Staff, in particular nurses, perceived PLWH as yearning for greater involvement in decision making than PLWH themselves actually reported. The opposite was true for information-seeking, with PLWH reporting higher levels of need than staff perceived. PLWH with symptoms tended to report lower levels of autonomy than those who were well, suggesting that being unwell decreased the desire to be personally involved in decision-making.

The start of person-centred HIV care

In the early days of the HIV epidemic, PLWH and their professional carers had been brought together by the urgency and poor prognosis of the condition, and close relationships developed between PLWH and their professional carers, with patients being engaged in all aspects of their care, sharing in the limited knowledge of HIV and treatments available at the time. That the doctors could do little in terms of treatment, helped to create the foundation for a more balanced, rather than paternalistic relationship, where doctors could not hold all the power of insight into the patients' predicament. This appeared to be the case even when sick patients would expect their doctors to provide some guidance to alleviate their symptoms. As Weeks (2007, p102) has argued, "people with HIV and AIDS proved to be the harbingers of a profound shift in the relationship between medicine and society".

In contrast with the stigma and discrimination faced by people with AIDS in the outside world, the atmosphere in HIV specialist clinics and wards could feel to PLWH like a welcome haven. The provision of complementary therapies, like massage, reflexology, and acupuncture (which often went hand-in-hand with more holistic philosophies of health) provided by charities and volunteers helped to alleviate symptoms, and contributed to making the experience of being involved in hospital care less clinical and more about the person. In everyday practice, wards and clinics were reportedly characterised by a relaxed, friendly atmosphere, with doctors and nurses often being on first-name terms with their patients, and where volunteers had a presence providing additional practical support. These comments by a gay man living with HIV are characteristic of the experience:

> *Time, kindness and honesty from all, nurses, doctors, and psychologists, and a frank admission that there wasn't a treatment for HIV, only symptomatic treatments. We had a very good relationship with the doctors and nurses, even the domestic staff were friendly. And there were things that made you feel better, like massage and aromatherapy. When you are frightened, a kind and gentle touch is what you want.*

What led to the development of person-centred care in HIV?

"*We were led by them [the patients] in terms of what they wanted, we got to know them really well, we had long-term relationships with them*," as one female HIV nurse stated.

Early on, consultants from a range of specialties became interested in treating people with HIV. Many of these pioneers were highly motivated and committed individuals. They became attracted to caring for people with HIV for a variety of reasons, including the intellectual appeal of a new disease of unknown aetiology and with no known treatment, and the personal investment of caring for patients belonging to stigmatised populations (gay men, drug users) doubly stigmatised by HIV. The complexity of the difficulties faced by patients soon led to the formation of multidisciplinary teams. The intensity of the process of young people identifying with – and caring for – young people who were likely to die, seemed to bring fresh approaches and a determination to treat HIV patients well, as an HIV physician explained:

> *It was challenging because they were our age in the main, most of us were in our late 20s and early 30s, and they were people like us and they were getting very sick and dying, and that engendered a very strong camaraderie amongst the clinicians and the patients. We, the junior doctors, had the knowledge, as our bosses didn't know more than us, and that was a very healthy state of affairs, there was no considered wisdom, just a set of values and a desire to do better for patients. We were all in uncharted territory. We always kept the patient at the centre, we never lost the view that the patient was more important than the next paper or the hospital or anything, we knew that the patient was the centre of it.*

The horrific experience of dealing with young people presenting to hospital so seriously ill, emaciated, distressed, and often close to death, in the absence of effective treatments, led to changes in the relationship between doctors and nurses and their patients, helped by the ring-fenced funding that allowed the services to develop in less conventional ways (Bruton et al. 2019). When a charity worker referred to 'death as the magic ingredient', he was highlighting the powerful impact of the overwhelming situation faced by PLWH and the doctors and nurses looking after them, which challenged not only the biomedical paradigm, but also the very foundations of health professionals' lives. The development of relationships, and recognition of the humanity of 'the other' was a powerful factor shaping the development of health professionals working in the field, as described by an HIV physician:

> *Most people died with tremendous courage, and it was a terrible time, in that we really had no available treatments. All we could really do was make people die in dignity. So, in the early phase it was very stressful but with a very strong sense of community as well. A whole new world opened to me, of different relationships and of different ways of people thinking and different activities and what people were doing with their lives, and it became a very fascinating thing. We produced one of the first, I think, really genuinely multidisciplinary approaches to management.*

For many nurses, the focus on dealing with end of life matters became paramount, including working with partners and families in the process. Again, the experience had strong resonance beyond the purely clinical aspects, becoming personally meaningful in sometimes profound ways, as told by this gay male nurse:

> *The terminal care experience was very important for us nurses and for the doctors, the drive to make it a good death was very powerful. There were great difficulties around supporting families who were struggling, supporting people who were gay or drug users. It was an immense privilege to be involved, I think it gave our lives more meaning, it gave a huge meaning to life and to understanding what was precious about it, it made the experience very special.*

Not only were health professionals recognising the humanity of patients, but the personal qualities of doctors and nurses involved in the care of people with HIV were recognised by PLWH. They frequently saw them as committed pioneers responding to a major health crisis, and who were co-developing with them something that would later be called person-centred care. A gay man living with HIV described his experience of being looked after by such healthcare professionals in glowing terms:

> *There was a group of nurses that you could only describe as fantastic, absolutely dedicated. They knew all they could do was to try to make people comfortable and prepare them for what was coming, because we were all told by then that we were dying. The doctors were incredible, we used first names, the whole new model of patient–doctor*

relationship began to form, dealing holistically with the person. I think it was probably the first time in the NHS history that people were in teams and worked as teams to try and help us out, not patronising you, not talking over you.

A majority of those presenting with symptoms of AIDS were young, articulate, white, and middle class, many of whom had been directly involved in the highly effective gay liberation activism that had emerged post Stonewall (Armstrong and Crage 2006). As such, they were able to make their needs and wishes understood, and this had the effect of offsetting the inherent power that resided in medical and nursing teams. The fact that PLWH faced stigma and rejection added to the feeling that they were entitled to be heard – and they were, as documented by this gay man:

It was the power of the group, the power of the people, particularly articulate gay men who were at the forefront of the first wave of the epidemic, and we were antsy, we were angry, we knew how to get organised, and we knew how to get what we wanted.

The political landscape of the time was also relevant, with a mixture of social conservatism and the start of decades of neoliberal economics to come, which meant that healthcare workers would choose a political position that supported better care and further planning of services, as was hinted by an activist living with HIV:

The context in the '80s was very divisive politics and you had a few doctors, who tended to be young and who were from different disciplines that included GU medicine, who actually saw beyond what was happening and how impossible as a medical problem this new condition was. And they slowly built specialised services that were able to provide some reasonable shelter from the nightmare that was going on outside.

However, it was not a straightforward and seamless path towards developing the HIV patient-centred model. Activists described their struggles to change attitudes, especially amongst the older generation of clinicians and managers, and the importance of activists and young professionals in the formation of a different model of care.

I remember in the early days sitting on a health authority AIDS advisory committee and talking about testing, and a lot of doctors saying, no, people don't want to know, we don't need to ask them if they want to be tested – we challenged a lot of preconceptions, the paternalism thing – it created a space in which a group of 'articulate patients' could come along and in a sense fill the space, and medical professionals had to listen because they needed our knowledge.

Volunteers began to establish a presence on the wards and clinics, finding ways of demonstrating their skills and commitment to the more open-minded clinicians. Peer input itself subsequently became important, and began to resonate in relation to chronic or severe diseases other than HIV. A younger generation of doctors were particularly open to working differently, some from the same communities affected by HIV, and began to make an impact on the development of services. A gay activist with HIV commented on what was happening at the time:

> *At first it was difficult to provide help in the hospital as a volunteer, because of the physician-centred model and the resistance of physicians to sharing and allowing any help at all – so we had to start working with younger doctors who were more open to the idea that medicine isn't solely the domain of the medics, but this changed later when deaths on the wards became overwhelming, and there was then a willingness to collaborate with the community and allow it to provide services on the wards.*

Charities providing end of life care, such as the London Lighthouse, developed unique models of care focusing on the centrality of the person with HIV (Cantacuzino 1993; Spence 1996), that proved inspirational for the HIV care sector beyond the charities. A charity worker perceptively referred to the role of charities in advancing the delivery of care:

> *I think when new ground is broken, it is often broken by the voluntary sector, before the statutory sector gets it – I think the integrated model of care was ahead in the voluntary sector in HIV – I think the statutory health and social services sector relies more on the rhetoric of empowerment then the reality.*

The process of identification with their patients was a strong component of the development of the patient–professional relationship. Apart from the similarities in age and gender, for gay and lesbian doctors and nurses, their sexuality was a significant factor in their choice of work and commitment. A female nurse commented on this process:

> *There was a lot of homophobia in nursing generally, male nurses automatically thought of as gay, and so for gay male nurses working in HIV was about being able to do something for their community.*

A gay male nurse dealing with his own internalised homophobia at the time illustrated the power of gay relationships on the hospital wards. He described watching a gay man on the ward devotedly looking after his dying partner. The open display of love between them blew apart the negative messages he had previously taken on board about homosexuality being unacceptable:

> *He wouldn't even go to the toilet and leave him, and of course the message was that being gay wasn't wrong. I knew gay people could love each other, but I'd never seen love like it. That was a very positive message to give a gay man who was a bit closeted. Oh my God, all those messages about being gay were all wrong.*

Identification worked in other ways too. For example, one physician who looked after injecting drug users began to realise that some patients shared the same working-class background with him:

I came from very similar social background to my patients, working-class background, nobody had been to university in my family. The patients were poor and I knew what it was like to be like that, and I suppose I did identify with them.

Recognition of the stigma suffered by people with AIDS and a strong determination to fight it, added a moral and political dimension to the process of caring for them. One doctor was so motivated by his moral outrage at negative public attitudes that he became even more determined to stay in the field and do as much as possible to help:

I don't think, one didn't think, about not doing it, why would one? It was interesting, it was challenging, and I felt very offended by public attitudes. So, I felt, well, you had better stay in there and try to make it better. I don't think I ever thought about not doing it – or anybody I worked with. I felt really angry that society behaved in a way that I found sad, unsympathetic and stigmatising of a group who couldn't necessarily help that they were infected. I became in a sense much more angry about it and motivated.

Dealing with HIV stigma could sometimes happen at a symbolic level, facilitated by the intimacy and closeness that grew between doctors, nurses, and their patients. A powerful example was given by a nurse who described how sharing a meal with a bedridden man with AIDS created a connection that powerfully challenged stigma:

I remember this guy on the ward who had some food wrapped in tin foil that somebody had brought him, and when he unwrapped it, I said, oh that looks nice, trying to make conversation. He then said, would you like some, and I said oh yes, and took a little bit, and he looked up and his eyes were full of tears. I realised he was upset because I had shared his food, he was used to being treated like a leper.

Intimacy outside the clinical setting was sometimes a consequence of the newer and less rigid relationships between PLWH and their doctors and nurses. A breaking down of barriers between patients and professionals became a defining characteristic of the field. An HIV physician reported on out-of-hospital interactions:

We were a big team and on Friday nights 65 or 70 people would go to the pub over the road for a drink, and the patients would pop in, and they were welcome. After closing time, we would sometimes go to the local gay club, and you just said, "I'm a doctor at the HIV unit and these are my mates," and you were let in straight away.

Lessons for the healthcare workers

The model of care that nurses and doctors co-developed with patients resulted in changes in the way they practised, both in terms of the informality of the exchanges and the organisation of the clinical services. In general, it seemed that existing hierarchies were being challenged to the extent that greater equality was inevitable between the professions and with patients, as described here by an HIV nurse:

> *I had been trained at a hospital which was quite traditional, but when I started working at the HIV ward, that's where I properly learnt to be a nurse; there was this amazing feeling of camaraderie, you could move mountains with it, there was a flattened hierarchy, we were all in it together.*

The message that patients had taught the nurses how to become true professionals was frequently mentioned, showing the two-way benefits between staff and patients of a shared partnership. A community nurse talked about her experience and the lessons she learnt:

> *I learnt a lot – I had been bossy and organised, but I learnt to support the patients' choice, that's what these patients taught me, it changed me. I have never felt that passion in any other area of work.*

The more informal ward rounds and other clinical meetings would sometimes give permission to even the most junior members of the team to speak-up more, and develop a sense of confidence in their own abilities and capacity to learn from complex clinical situations. A young female nurse recalled her work on the ward:

> *It wasn't rigid, it was very fluid because we were patient centred, patient focused, and as a newly qualified staff nurse it was a really good environment. Doctors and nurses, we all worked together, you didn't need to be frightened to ask a question which in other specialties, when you were quite low on the rung of your career life, you were very hesitant in asking something if you didn't understand.*

It seemed a creative and welcoming environment for young people with ideas, aspirations, and concerns about human rights, partly because HIV infection was a new and stigmatised disease requiring new solutions, but also because of the way HIV medicine was separated out and allowed to thrive, away from the gaze of more conservative elements of the NHS. An HIV physician remembered the comparative openness of the clinical environment:

> *It was a young specialty, so not as stiff or traditional as cardiology or neurology. It was full of people who got there because they didn't feel they fitted into some of the more old-school methods, so it is quite innovative and dynamic – so not only did we have a huge diversity of patients but we had a huge diversity of staff, and people felt they could be themselves. We also benefited from being isolated from some of that, no one wanted to touch it, no one else really understood it, so you lot over there could deal with it.*

However, the closeness between PLWH and nurses and doctors led to porous boundaries that could introduce difficulties. Boundaries were sometimes difficult to navigate, and their management jarred with more traditional ways of behaving.

Traditionally, physical contact between professional carers and patients, apart from the obvious contact involved in physical examinations or in nursing and medical procedures, would be restricted perhaps to a handshake. In the case of HIV care, physical contact would often include more intimate expressions of support, such as hugging or hand holding. Apart from demonstrating concern for the patient, such acts were also a response to the prevailing stigmatisation of PLWH. A gay male nurse described some of the issues raised by closer physical contact:

> *Boundaries [were] an issue, some of the doctors on the ward were concerned about nurses who were hugging patients, there was a tension between reassuring somebody that he is not infectious, and the impact on the traditional service.*

Inevitably, the close bond between clinicians and PLWH could reach more intense and distressing levels when the latter were reaching the end of their lives. A high level of intimacy and engagement with a sick person with HIV over the last few weeks of that person's life could result in over involvement on the part of the nurse or the doctor, with obvious distress. There was also the possibility of risking or mismanaging the clinical aspects of care, by failing to keep enough distance. Exposure to multiple and repeated experiences of loss would test the psychological strength and resilience of the professional, as well as the solidity of the multidisciplinary team. A male HIV nurse recalled its impact:

> *The intensity of feeling and involvement in looking after dying patients of the same age as we were led to a real emotional intimacy between you and the patients, and I think that is partly why it took its toll on us as well. We should have protected ourselves better. But I wouldn't change it.*

There were attempts to manage the closeness of relations with patients. Hospices, for example, reported that rituals were introduced to deal with the frequent occurrence of death to help carers cope with the pain and sadness of the loss of somebody that had been the centre of care and attention, as remembered by a female nurse:

> *When somebody died, we made sure there was always somebody with them, and if they didn't have anybody, we would be with them. I have been with dozens of people when they died, holding their hands and just being there with them. We would always light a candle on the reception desk when somebody died, and sometimes when you came in there would be six candles. It was pretty heavy going.*

The 'one-stop shop'

Person-centred care developed with the involvement of patients in decision-making, together with a system of care where consultations with a range of relevant specialists took place by the bedside, and in outpatient and family clinics. Traditionally, referral to non-HIV specialists would have required a consultant to consultant referral, or a referral through the GP to the relevant specialist, thus delaying and prolonging the process of assessment and care.

In the case of HIV, an in-house system (or 'silo', according to critics) developed, providing an intimate circle of support and expertise, that also spilled over into life outside the clinic. Such developments were not planned in advance, but developed incrementally and organically, from ad hoc meetings, that were shaped by the input and experiences of patients. No doubt, this inclusive system was reinforced by the relative isolation that HIV specialists sometimes faced within the hospital community, which was related to the negative attitudes expressed towards certain patients such as gay men and so-called 'difficult patients', for example drug users. A physician working with drug users with HIV remembered this kind of development:

> *We grew the service gradually, using existing resources, and gradually widened and strengthened the team of doctors and nurses, we hired sessional doctors, clinical assistants, we started to get patients from other services, like maternity, many with medical complications, then we got dieticians, and then counselling – the psychiatrists weren't interested, there was no mental health drug service, they didn't want to prescribe methadone, what's the point, they will not give up drugs – so us on the ward first, and some GPs after discharge did it – it was a battle at first.*

The 'one-stop shop' was not restricted to hospital wards or outpatient clinics. The model was extended to the links with palliative care and its extension to the community, which sometimes led to the inclusion of active treatment. A physician working with drug users described the process of adapting practice to the patients' needs:

> *The charity was set up for terminal care, widening it to improve quality of life, with ring-fenced funding, and they had access to homebased packages of care – it was an interesting shift from palliative care to home based care, with expert people managing it – we had multidisciplinary meetings discussing more aggressive treatments rather than just palliative care, we talked about people with the most complex needs – that is how the HIV model of care was grounded.*

In specialist HIV services, the provision of access to mental health care was an early development that included clinical psychologists, counsellors, and psychiatrists working very closely with the medical and nursing teams, in ways that many doctors had not experienced before. Clinical psychologists and other mental health specialists worked alongside the clinical teams, seeing patients on the wards and clinics, and sharing information and care plans. A clinical psychologist described her multiple roles:

> *The role of the clinical psychologist was to support the person with HIV in the clinic and on the dedicated HIV ward that had just opened, we provided continuity of care as people were diagnosed, went in, were discharged, came in again etc – you knew the doctors and the nurses involved well, and the rest of the team, and you could be involved in coordinating care, deciding who did what.*

HIV person-centred care after 1996: is HIV a chronic manageable condition?

The development of new and effective treatments and their widespread use led to major changes in the prognosis of HIV infection, with significant reductions in mortality and in HIV-associated medical problems. At the same time, changes occurred in the provisions of services, which adapted to the new landscape of HIV illness, and later were influenced by wider political change.

Towards the end of the 1990s, the concept of HIV infection as a chronic manageable condition started to be talked about by clinicians and researchers. The concept was however questioned from the outset because of the unduly optimistic message it gave, minimising the significance of the condition, and implying that a cure had been found that kept the disease at bay, while many PLWH continued to experience significant health problems. What was always a long-term condition with a bad prognosis, remained a chronic condition with a better prognosis, but often with continued multiple associated chronic health problems and ongoing stigma (Catalan et al. 2001; Goldman 2001). As reported by the National AIDS Trust (2016), the vast majority of PLWH have at least one other medical condition, and almost a third, three or more health problems. While for some PLWH the term 'chronic manageable condition' was seen as a positive way of normalising HIV, for others it was perceived as a rebranding that tended to ignore not just the importance of added physical disorders, but also the psychological consequences and stigma still associated with HIV infection. As it has been said before, patients diagnosed with diabetes would not be reassured by being told, "Don't worry, your condition is just a chronic one, like HIV infection". A charity worker remembered the response of a PLWH:

> One of my patients was so offended when told his HIV was like diabetes now. "Yes," he said, "my CD4 may be good, but what about all my symptoms, my morbidities – diarrhoea, fatigue, constant battle with social services over money and benefits, and having to prove to others what my CD4 is, but my quality of life is ignored." It is the whole system they feel let down by.

The chronic and manageable concept potentially limits the range of options available within a person-centred model. If HIV is now like other chronic disorders, why should there be specialist services, such as mental health facilities for PLWH, rather than expecting patients to access generic services? A psychiatrist working with PLWH reported on referrals to specialist mental health teams:

> Since the 2000s, there has been an increase in the proportion of people referred suffering from depression, the problem is how to live, and how to make sense of the chronic condition, while trying to normalise their lives, relationships, and employment, with added unresolved problems accumulated over the years. There is pressure to refer such PLWH to the already overwhelmed generic mental health community services, that may not have the capacity or expertise required.

This process of 'normalisation', making HIV like other chronic conditions, has been seen as a justification for the decline in the level of person-centred care provided to PLWH, with a loss of continuity and consistency. 'Normalisation' would for some mean that HIV care would possibly be as poor as that available for other chronic diseases. In the words of an HIV activist:

> It is sometimes argued that we are trying to make HIV a special case, when other chronic, serious disorders don't need such care, but the point to make is that we should not provide HIV patients with the lowest common denominator level of care, just because that is what other patients get: we should try to raise the care of other conditions to the level of care we endeavour to provide in HIV.

Adapting to the stresses and strains of change

The well-established HIV person-centred model of care continued to be regarded as the gold standard by PLWH and their professional carers, but there were important changes in its focus and in its delivery. The development of effective antiretroviral treatments, some involving complex regimens and unpleasant side-effects, focused the attention of PLWH and their doctors on medication. As a result, changes took place in the interaction between PLWH and their professional carers. A senior HIV doctor went as far as to highlight a major alteration in the delivery of care:

> So, there was a big shift away from the patient being at the centre of care to the drugs being at the centre.

Balancing models of care, from the person-centred without effective treatment model of earlier times, to the model that requires decisions about different treatment regimens, discussion of side-effects, and treatment adherence, while striving to keep the PLWH at the centre of decision-making, became an important shift, and one that at times was difficult for people with HIV and doctors to navigate. This shift in focus also meant that doctors acquired greater pharmacological knowledge than the majority of PLWH, a significant change from the 'shared ignorance' of the earlier days. A gay man living with HIV remembered the change:

> In those early days the only model that was going to work was one of partnership – there was so much stigma, there was no treatment, so you needed this partnership – people diagnosed later go back to a different doctor–patient relationship: you are diagnosed, you take these pills, off you go, bang.

The growth in pharmacological information about effective drug combinations, drug interactions, and adverse side-effects led to a change in the balance of knowledge and expertise between and within professional carers and PLWH, creating a new hierarchy of knowledge, as a nurse remembered:

> The divisions between doctors, patients, and nurses grew larger because of knowledge about drugs, then I think patients lost a bit of their voice – oh, it has become a chronic condition, so there is no need to fight.

The demand for continuation of a truly person-centred approach was made by HIV charities and PLWH who had been involved in the development of the original models of care. For some PLWH, a new sense of mistrust and bitterness crept in, with blame directed at the new doctors and nurses for showing what was claimed to be a poor attitude to their care, although this view did not seem to be widespread among PLWH. A gay man living with HIV, however, recalled the shift in behaviour:

> *There was this golden era of maybe a decade … HIV became the model for others to emulate and copy, but funding and politics, and I think other things, was the original pioneers that came to the call got exhausted and moved on, and then the careerists moved in, and the ambitious doctors and nurses moved in and wanted to make a career out of our misery – they don't want antsy patients telling them what to do, and that's when things began to change.*

For other PLWH, the changes reflected a political dimension that impacted on the provision of care:

> *The sense of intense crisis was changing, and then you got this separation and fragmentation again, and the recreation of silos against an economic context of increasing neoliberalism, which was also about managerialism and atomisation once the pills came along, the government said, well, we don't need to fund so much now, and also we had a strengthening of the neoliberal model which says, right if you want money you need to compete for it, and then you end up moving towards a monopoly, which is what happened in the charity sector.*

The widespread use of effective antiretroviral drugs had important consequences for hospital and charity-based services. On the one hand, there was less of a need for inpatient or hospice beds, and on the other hand, outpatient clinics became much busier. The reduction in bed usage, while welcome, led to a dilution of continuity of care in some services, which in itself was perceived as having a negative effect. A physician regretted some of the changes that followed:

> *Two things changed: first they said we didn't need so many beds, so they went; second, we lost continuity because patients were admitted under whoever was on call, and remained under that team for the duration of their stay – the loss of continuity of care was the main change.*

Pressures of work and sheer numbers of PLWH attending clinics, leading to a lessening of contact between nurses and PLWH played a part in the dissatisfaction expressed by some PLWH, nurses, and doctors. A nurse described some efforts to adapt the nurses' skills to the practice changes:

> *We were trying to widen the nurses' skills to become nurse practitioners, but we found that they were now much busier in clinics with so many patients who were now surviving, and they were spending time on basic tasks like taking bloods, and becoming*

deskilled, not able to talk to patients. So, we introduced health care assistants to take the less skilled jobs from the nurses, and leave them the more skilled ones.

Doctors too recognised that increased demands on them because of sheer numbers undermined their satisfaction with the care they were delivering:

Continuity is what made it work better. I think I was delivering personal care, and I preferred it when I had my group of patients to look after, rather than this great pyramid and when other people are looking after the patients you are technically responsible for.

Increasing uniformity of care was a source of regret for doctors who were used to a more flexible, person-tailored support, and who now felt under pressure to provide a more streamlined service, echoing the concerns expressed about 'managerialism' by the activist quoted above. Financial pressures and new management protocols contributed to this loss of flexibility:

We are losing individualisation of care. Junior doctors are much more under managerial control, and will be more likely to do as they are told. In the early days, patients would choose the doctor they wanted to see because of their style of care. Some would like to spend 40 minutes with the doctor, and would see that one, while others just wanted one minute, and would then make their choice. There is no right or wrong way to practise medicine, and I think the lack of individuality is actually having an impact on the level and degree of care.

What happened to the 'one-stop shop'?

A reduction in the numbers of people needing inpatient care and changes in their medical needs, led to changes in the established pattern of specialists attending joint clinics or sessions, and a return to more traditional appointments. An HIV physician described some of the shifts and their possible consequences:

The specialists found it was inefficient to come to see one or two patients at the HIV clinic, so patients were expected to go to the routine OP clinics of the specialist. There was a shift from patients being feared like the plague and being sent to the HIV team, to the idea that anybody can treat HIV probably making the quality of care less good.

Some degree of person-centred care became lost in the process of onward referrals, when the needs of the service seemed to take priority over those of the PLWH. A clinical psychologist reported on some of the developing strains:

Care for HIV and for all kinds of other illnesses went backwards in the sense that nothing could be coordinated at a local level to the best advantage of the patient. Patient care become disjointed and probably in the long run more expensive.

These views are echoed in the comments of a person who was living with HIV for many years, who reflected on the changes in the organisation of care:

> *I'd never want to wind the clock back on the disease, but I wouldn't have minded winding the clock so that the HIV clinic was the main point for everything and you would be referred out from there. You would just know that if you felt ill, that's where you would go.*

In earlier days, the one-stop shop model included those providing practical support, such as dietitians and social workers, the latter employed by the local authority, but frequently based with the HIV team. However, that dimension of care, which would have provided support for aspects of living, such as nutrition, adaptations to the home and financial benefits, became separated from the established team. An HIV physician regretted this loss:

> *As for social services, as soon as it moved into the community it lost the team approach – if you need a social worker, you must go to the town hall … while beforehand there would be social workers in house to sort things out – disintegration of the team approach.*

HIV person-centred care now

The relevance of the 'one-stop shop' model in relation to mental health is highlighted by further research from the US on the effect of expanding on-site mental health care services for PLWH. Aggarwal et al. (2019) showed that such a move led to better HIV outcomes, with viral suppression increasing from 57% to 88%, and to a greater number of patients being found to have substance misuse diagnoses. Another study of a large cohort of almost 6,000 participants, showed pharmacological treatment of psychiatric disorders in PLWH to be associated with viral suppression (Levy et al. 2019).

The success of ART in reducing HIV-related morbidity and mortality, and the subsequent move from mainly inpatient to predominantly outpatient care, and the change in delivery of care from a 'one-stop shop' to more traditional clinical care, contributed to the shift away from provision of care in specialist centres. Less needed were the highly experienced and committed nurses and doctors, as local GPs – usually less experienced in the care of PLWH – took over care of PLWH.

While these changes in the care of HIV were in many ways a creative and understandable response to the evolving condition, they nevertheless continue to be contested today. With the majority of PLWH now primarily being cared for by their GP, there are mixed reviews. Additionally, maintaining person-centred care here is specially challenging, as a gay man living with HIV articulated:

> *There has been a weakening of the patient-centred model in HIV, as patients are seen less frequently, and their needs are supposed to be taken care of by the GP. While some GPs are very good and patients are comfortable with them, and they keep a*

good relationship with the HIV medics, there is a perception amongst patients that GPs are too busy and not sufficiently confident to identify what is HIV related and what isn't.

Another direct consequence of the changes to service delivery and disease progression can be seen in the changed relationship between PLWH and their specialist carers. A charity worker reflected on then and now, and concluded relationships had to adapt:

What is different too is the nature of the relationships we developed with people who we expected would die soon. If you are looking after somebody in the last months of his life, the closeness is not the same when you see somebody doing well every six months. Those earlier relationships would be regarded as inappropriate by many today.

The relationship between HIV specialist services and general practice

An important change, following the reduction in need for inpatient care with a parallel increase in outpatient and community support, has been the reappraisal of the role of the general practitioner in HIV care, from testing to the provision of continued, routine HIV care. HIV physicians appreciate the need for changes in the delivery of HIV care as the majority of PLWH require less frequent input from an HIV specialist now. However, questions remain about how best to ensure that optimum and accessible care for PLWH continues to be available, as raised by an HIV physician:

We have been very lucky that patients can still have direct access to secondary services without having to go through the GP … but with new commissioning arrangements it is going to be more difficult for people to choose what clinic they want to go to.

PLWH, particularly those used to the earlier model of care based in specialist HIV centres, are less happy with these changes, citing concerns which include the possible loss of confidentiality about their HIV infection and their sexuality, and fears of overt and covert discrimination. A charity worker commented on the complex dilemmas facing clinical services:

The room for service redesign is immense. Does it mean that HIV care should be moved from the specialist centres into primary care? There are many people with HIV who would absolutely fight against that, all the way. There are many vested interests within hospitals that want to keep it there. But is it a good use of PLWH's time to go a long distance to a consultant, a high-cost setting when it is not really necessary anymore? The case load of clinics has rocketed, but should they be there in the first place? Have we protected services to the detriment of what would actually work better at a community level for people who are going to be long-term NHS users?

Those arguing for the greater involvement of GPs in the care of PLWH frequently suggest that GPs are better placed to monitor the co-morbidities that develop as PLWH become older and/or present with more advanced disease. It is also argued that treating PLWH in regular general practice appointments is less stigmatising than treating them in a special and, to some extent, concealed way. These were the views of one HIV physician:

> We used to have the silo model where we dealt with everything, but I do not think that is the right way forward now for a chronic condition, which HIV is. It allows stigma to persist, it allows ignorance to persist, it allows incompetence to persist. I think people with HIV need to go down the same pathway of care for their cancer or cardiovascular disease, or mental health problems, and they need to involve primary care. I think it is a disservice if they don't. Resistance to this idea comes from professionals and from patients. Some professionals don't want to give up their role, but as with other diseases you need a general practitioner as much as a specialist, and they need to talk to each other. The model of care needs to continue to evolve.

PLWH, especially those who have had a long history of contact with their HIV specialists, have concerns about the loosening of the association with them, even when the arguments for greater closeness with primary care are understood.

> I only have contact with my HIV consultant every six months or so, and I have a very longstanding relationship with him, I have full confidence in him and have little need of care. Ageing means that I need to be monitored for a number of potential conditions, and it involves me travelling long distances for various scans and it takes a day, so the alternative would be to go to another and closer HIV centre, but I would miss the special relationship with my consultant and the expertise of the hospital. I have a good GP but shared care hasn't really been tested yet.

Organisational changes of this kind raise important questions about this model of care. Are there limits to a person-centred care model in this new world? Does it still cater for the needs and wishes of PLWH, rather than service needs? Who makes the treatment decisions now? A heterosexual man living with HIV expressed his concerns:

> One size doesn't fit all. You can say to a guy in his 20s or 30s, I will see you in six months, and they will go, fine – but for someone in their 60s to say come back in six months, I don't think that is appropriate. I think there should be more monitoring for people who need the reassurance, not just the physical reassurance but also the mental support of keeping contact with the clinic.

The ability to make treatment choices with access to expert advice on HIV if needed, is recognised as essential by PLWH, as it has clear consequences for their health, as outlined by a gay man living with HIV:

*I think the range of solutions that the healthcare system can offer has expanded enor-
mously. My experience has been rather privileged, attending an excellent London clinic,
where people knew everything that there was to know about HIV. If I had been living
elsewhere, relying on my local GP, I think I would have had a rather different experience. That variety of knowledge and experience is probably still there across the health
system as a whole.*

PLWH repeatedly questioned the need for this shift in the organisation of their
care, sometimes feeling that they have lost the kind of care they had struggled to
achieve. They regretted that the care available could no longer be viewed as person-centred care in the way that it once was:

*I don't understand why care has been moved to GPs, I really don't. It's for structural
benefit. I think lots of my stuff could be done in the HIV clinic, all the regular boring
stuff could be done with a GP, it always seemed easier to have a GP in the HIV clinic
than me going to the health centre and explaining every time to a different GP. They
are good and they are interested but they know nothing about HIV, and I have to
explain everything. There is a lot of confusion about what constitutes treatment for HIV
and what for non-HIV condition. It is definitely not beneficial to the patients. We
weren't spoilt, we had the care we fought for.*

The impact of wider changes to health care provision is illustrated by the situation
in England following the Health and Social Care Act 2012. The change led to
separation of the financing and organisation of sexual health services and prevention, from the financing and organisation of HIV specialist care. Thus, integration
of these prevention and care services was no longer a priority for the provider.
Even amongst GPs, there is concern about both their willingness and ability to deal
with HIV, on top of all the other pressures they face in their day-to-day work. An
experienced GP, working in an area where injecting drug use is prevalent, recognised the complexities introduced by the Act:

*Being a GP, I think GPs are the centre of the universe, and I think we can do things
across most sectors and we have a setup, local provision, local medical facilities, we have
nursing, doctors, health visitors, care of children, social work on site. So, we have a broad
provision for primary care, but the new generation of GPs is completely not interested,
completely not interested, and it is worse in England because the Lansley ghastly bill
has taken drugs out of the NHS, and in the hands of local authorities, so the local
authorities are struggling with this, trying to manage drug users, and on top of that, we
have private health care providers setting up clinics, top slicing money from the NHS to
fund them.*

The complexity of the combined effects of political and practical changes, economic factors, varying levels of expertise, and services split between HIV specialists
and GPs are difficult for anyone fully to comprehend. Amongst other uncertainties,
there is a question mark about what role, if any, the PLWH has in this new context.

An experienced charity worker questioned a range of assumptions made when introducing new approaches to care:

> *On the other hand, there are GP stories, HIV is far too complicated and expensive, so we don't want it. So, at what point do we want overstretched primary care doctors to start prescribing antiretrovirals, is that a better way of doing it? What are the economics of it? Do we risk losing the centres of excellence that drive continued clinical trials? What about when treatment stops working? What about complex cases? So, it isn't a simple matter of let's move into primary care. It is really complex stuff. But we haven't grasped it properly. Is there the will amongst clinicians and the leading community activists to drive forward the next stage of change?*

Aspirations and hurdles in the continuation of person-centred HIV care

In early 2016, the National AIDS Trust (NAT) organised a national conference to discuss the drivers of change in HIV care, identify difficulties for HIV long-term condition management, and to set up an agenda for future policy. The published report (NAT, 2016), detailed the fundamentals of HIV care that needed to be maintained, such as the meaningful engagement of PLWH in all areas of service reform, access to the most appropriate medication for meeting an individual's needs, and open access for all to HIV services. The report made it clear that this essential care is frequently not in place. Furthermore, the report stressed the need to integrate HIV services with HIV-competent primary care, something that will require much more than good intentions. NAT's findings resonate with those concerns of many people we interviewed for this book.

The NAT report also highlighted the requirement for person-centred care, in line with NHS England's commitment to this model of care (NHS England, 2015). Suggestions included the development of Positive Self-Management programmes, such as the Expert Patients Programme. Some good examples of patient involvement are already in existence, as described by a patient representative working in one of London's HIV clinics:

> *We have three paid patient representatives, we run workshops, newly diagnosed courses, forums, hepatitis workshops, women's lunch club, a choir, and do special events. It is very powerful to talk to people recently diagnosed and say to them, look I have been positive for 30 years. We are able to access medical records now, and we can help the doctors. We provide continuity.*

The London based independent think tank, The King's Fund, subsequently published a report that focused on the future organisation of HIV services in England, including HIV prevention as well as care for those already infected (Baylis et al. 2017). Its conclusions are consistent with those cited in the NAT (2016) publication. This report highlighted the need for local and national bodies to work together with HIV stakeholders, in the context of the Health and Social Care Act 2012 and the financial austerity that is affecting local authority budgets. Much attention is given to the implications for care with the involvement of both GPs and other specialist services, and to the concerns of PLWH about the lack of service planning. Recommendations include reintegrating fragmented services, aligning HIV services and wider health policy, and planning for future models of care. The involvement of PLWH and other stakeholders is assumed in this report, which recognises the complexity of the tasks required to maintain and develop further high-quality HIV services. An example of the impact of financial austerity and its effects on person-centred care was given by a senior HIV physician:

> *Funding is the next big challenge. The cost of branded drugs is excessive and generics are now coming in, so it will mean that patients will not have a chance to choose what drug they will take.*

Quality of HIV care is the theme of a newer BHIVA publication, 'Standards of Care for People Living with HIV' (2018). BHIVA is a well-regarded organisation of UK HIV healthcare professionals, established in 1995, that focuses on the promotion of good practice in the treatment of HIV and public education, as well as dissemination of research. This comprehensive report aimed to provide a benchmark for the quality of HIV care. The importance of person-centred care is highlighted throughout, focusing on stigma, self-management, and peer support, together with the participation of PLWH in their care. A remarkable feature of the report is how each one of these topics contains a comprehensive list of quality standards, each with measurable and auditable outcomes, which would allow monitoring of the degree to which each goal has been achieved. In the case of person-centred care, both decisions about individual treatment and care, and the planning of services, are included as essential elements in the links between PLWH and their professional carers. In practice, person-centred HIV care is not always straightforward; it is not simply about giving the patients what they demand, but a process requiring negotiation between patient and clinical expertise, with the development of a shared awareness of the best available research evidence, and exploration of the person's perspectives, including priorities, goals, values and wishes (Barber et al. 2018).

Lessons from the person-centre HIV care model

The early development of HIV care is a unique example of the organic development of a person-centred model of care, which those interviewed for this book outlined in detail, highlighting its various elements and showing how it could work in practice. While it was not the first time that this personalised and integrated model of care had been advocated on such a large scale (e.g. see Ottawa Charter for Health Promotion, 1986), its practical implementation and the heights of sophistication it developed can be recognised as one of the positive outcomes from what was in many ways a tragic period in the history of health care in the UK. A senior HIV physician summed up the ground-breaking achievement in this way:

What you have loosely called patient-centred outcome is probably the best model there is, deciding what the patients want and what are their priorities and then providing that, rather than a doctor-centric model where the doctor decides what's best for the patients. I think patient involvement has been fairly revolutionary.

For many doctors and nurses, who during their training and in later practice aspired to a form of medicine which included patients as fundamental to shared decision-making, this approach became an example of how it could be achieved in practice. For some, this "holistic approach to the care of people with illnesses may be the most important lesson that HIV can teach medicine" (Catalan 1994).

While more research is needed into the delivery of person-centred care across care transitions, such as the move from inpatient to outpatient care (Santana et al. 2018; Backman and Cho-Young 2019), research into its effects in general medical conditions has shown the value of person-centred care in terms of containing healthcare costs, improving patient–clinician interactions, treatment adherence, and health outcomes (Stewart et al. 2014). Similarly, in the case of HIV care, preliminary research shows the value of this model of care in terms of patient engagement and better coordination of care (Ojikuto et al. 2014; Boyd and Lucas 2014; Cook et al. 2018; Wood et al. 2018; Wachira et al. 2018).

Conclusion

To what extent could the person-centred model of care have developed in the absence of HIV infection? It is true that currently there are repeated calls for such an approach in the practice of medicine in the UK, from NHS England (2015) and clinicians and researchers (Richards et al. 2013; Leng et al. 2017; Nolte 2017; de Iong et al. 2019), and it is quite likely that this shift in perspective away from the power of the clinician towards a collaborative approach would have occurred. However, what is significant is how much HIV care anticipated – and then became the forerunner of – the subsequent development of these models of care. As a gay male activist living with HIV expressed:

> *That change in paternalism was probably happening already but the whole idea that in order to understand patients in a way which enabled you to give the best care and support and treatment, you had to involve them and listen to them, and it changed this relationship from not just treating the disease in the person, but actually talking to the person. I think HIV gave a huge thrust to that, and it has spread beyond HIV.*

Documents like the NAT 2016 report and, in particular, the BHIVA (2018) 'Standards of Care for People Living with HIV' confirm how person-centred HIV care became the defining paradigm for PLWH and their professional carers. What remains to be seen is the extent of political will to guarantee the continuation of this model not just for HIV care, and not just as a rhetoric for medical conditions, but for all medical care in actuality.

References

Aggarwal R, Pham M, Dillingham R, McManus KA (2019) Expanded HIV clinic-based Mental Health Care Services: association with viral suppression. *Open Forum Infectious Diseases*, 6 (4), ofz146. DOI: 10.1093/ofid/ofz146.

Armstrong EA and Crage SM (2006) Movements and memory: the making of the Stonewall myth. *American Sociological Review*, 71(5), 724–751.

Backman C and Cho-Young D (2019) Engaging patients and informal caregivers to improve safety and facilitate person- and family-centered care during transitions from hospital to home. *Patient Preference and Adherence*, 13: 617–626.

Balint E (1969) The possibilities of patient-centred medicine. *Journal of the Royal College of General Practitioners*, 17: 269–276.

Barber T, Saunders JM, Barnett N (2018) Person-centred care and HIV: challenges and solutions. *Sexually Transmitted Infections*, 94: 582–584.

Baylis A, Buck D, Anderson J, Jabbal J and Ross S (2017) *The future of HIV services in England: shaping the response to changing needs.* London, The King's Fund.

BHIVA (2018) *Standards of Care for People Living with HIV.* ISBN: 978–0–9551669-6-9. London, Mediscript Ltd.

Bower P and Mead N (2007) Patient-centred healthcare. In Ayers S, Baum A, McManus C, Newman S, Wallston K, Weinman J, West R (eds) *Cambridge Handbook of Psychology, Health and Medicine.* Cambridge, Cambridge University Press.

Boyd CM and Lucas GM (2014) Patient-centred care for people living with multimorbidity. *Current Opinion HIV AIDS*, 9(4): 419–427.

Bruton J, Edwards S and Perry N (2019) The impact of AIDS on the traditional roles of UK healthcare workers and the emergence of new models of care. *AIDS IMPACT XIV International Conference*, July 29–31, London.

Cantacuzino M (1993) *Till break of day.* London, Heineman.

Carretero MD, Chiswick A, and Catalan J (1998) Whose health is it? The views of injecting drug users with HIV infection and their professional carers. *AIDS CARE*, 10, 3, 323–328.

Catalan J (1994) 'The doctor's tale'. In *Cry Love, Cry Hope*, Bill Kirkpatrick (ed), Darton, Longman and Todd Ltd., London.

Catalan J, Brener N, Andrews H, Day A, Cullum S, Hooker M, and Gazzard B (1994) Whose health is it? Views about decision-making and information-seeking from people with HIV infection and their professional carers. *AIDS CARE*, 6(3), 349–356.

Catalan J, Green L, Thorley F (2001) The changing picture of HIV: a chronic illness, again? *Focus: a guide to AIDS research and counselling*, 16(3) 1–4.

Cook CL, Canidate S, Ennis N, Cook RL (2018) Types and delivery of emotional support to promote linkage and engagement in HIV care. *Patience Preference and Adherence*, 12: 45–52.

de Iong A, Redding D, Leonard H (2019) New personalised care plan for the NHS. *British Medical Journal*, 364, 262.

Ende J, Kazis L, Ash A and Moskowitz M (1989) Measuring patients' desire for Autonomy. *Journal of General Internal Medicine*, 4, 23–30.

Goldman R (2001) Being chronically ill. *Focus: a guide to AIDS research and counselling*, 16, 3, 5–6.

Leng G, Ingham C, Brian K, Partridge G (2017) National Commitment to shared decision making. *British Medical Journal*, 359, 264.

Levy M, Monroe A, Horberg M, Benator D, Molock S, Doshi R, Happ L and Castle A (2019) Pharmacological treatment of psychiatric disorders and time with unsuppressed HIV viral load in a clinical HIV cohort. *Journal of Acquired Immune Deficiency Syndrome*, 82, 3, 329–341.

NAT (2016) *HIV in the future NHS: what next for people living with HIV in England.* www.nat.org.uk/publications

NAT (2017) *No-one left behind: a declaration on 'Whole person Care in HIV care and support'.* www.nat.org.uk/publications

NHS England (2015) *Our Declaration: Person-centred Care for Long Term-conditions.* https://www.england.nhs.uk/wp-content/uploads/2015/09/ltc-our-declaration.pdf

Nolte E (2017) Implementing person centred approaches. *British Medical Journal*, 358, 474.

Ojikuto B, Holman J, Kunches L, Landers S, Perlmutter D, Ward M, Fant G, Hirschhorn L (2014) Interdisciplinary HIV care in a changing healthcare environment in the USA. *AIDS CARE*, 26(6) 731–735.

Ottawa Charter for Health Promotion (1986) *The move towards a new public health. First International Conference for Health Promotion*, Ottawa, Ontario, Canada.

Richards T, Montori VM, Godlee F, Lapsley P, Paul D (2013) Let the patient revolution begin. *British Medical Journal*, 346, 7.

Roper N, Logan WW and Tierney AJ (2000) *The Roper-Logan-Tierney Model of Nursing.* Edinburgh, Elsevier Health Sciences.

Santana MJ, Manalili K, Jolley RJ, Zelinsky S, Quan H and Lu M (2018) How to practice person-centred care: a conceptual framework. *Health Expectations*, 21: 429–440. DOI: 10.1111/hex.12640

Spence C (1996) *On Watch: Views from the Lighthouse.* London, Cassell.

Stewart M, Brown JB, Weston WW, McWhinney IR, McWilliam CL, and Freeman TR. (2014) *Patient-centered medicine: transforming the clinical method.* (Third edition) London, CRC Press, Taylor & Francis.

Wachira J, Genberg B, Kafu C, Braitstein P, Laws MB, Wilson IB (2018) Experiences and expectations of patients living with HIV on their engagement with care in Western Kenya. *Patient Preference and Adherence*, 12: 1393–1400.

Weeks J (2007) *The World We Have Won.* London, Routledge.

Wood TJ, Koester KA, Christopoulos KA, Sauceda JA, Neilands TB, Johnson MO (2018) If someone cares about you, you are more apt to come around: improving HIV care engagement by strengthening the patient-provider relationship. *Patience Preference and Adherence*, 12: 919–927.

7   The changing narratives of HIV death and dying

Introduction

Tombstones and frightening icebergs forecasting death were part of the images linked with AIDS in the early days, leading to an association between infection and death in the public's mind, no doubt reflecting the reality of this link (Shilts 1987; Garfield 1994; Nuland 1994). Activists and policy makers found ways to develop networks of support and to guard against the worst kinds of discrimination affecting people with HIV. Residential services for palliative and terminal care established innovative models of holistic care (Cantacuzino 1993; Spence 1996). Specialist HIV units dealt with the ravages of advanced HIV infection as best they could. Similarly, in the US, the famous 'Denver Principles', drafted in 1983 by the People with AIDS Self-Empowerment Movement's advisory committee, identified the right of people living with HIV (PLWH) to be "active and equal partners in the response to HIV and AIDS" (Morolake, Stephens, and Welbourn 2009; King 2013).

Many ill people were of similar age and background to those looking after them, contributing to a strong emotional connection between patients and care teams, enlightening healthcare workers, and involving them in their lives in ways that other patients had not before. The awareness of death led to many instances of open conversations about 'living wills', and to the planning of funerals as celebrations of the lives of those that had died. The concept of 'death literacy' (Spence 1996) was introduced to highlight the inevitable familiarity with death that was required during these times. The large number of deaths among previously healthy young men (Rosenfeld, Bartlam, and Smith 2012) became part of the public imagination. AIDS quilts, panels that movingly commemorated individuals who had died of AIDS, helped to bring AIDS to public attention. In the USA, the thousands of panels displayed in Washington in 1987 had increased fourfold by 1988 (Blair and Michel 2007).

Effective antiretroviral therapy (ART) (Hammer, Squires, Hughes et al. 1997), gradually reduced the incidence of death among people with HIV. An increasing sense of hope in survival led to a shift in the perception of HIV infection from a death sentence to a manageable condition. Eventually, survival became not just a possibility, but something likely. Palliative care was seen as less necessary, and some of the services that had been developed in the earlier phase of the epidemic became less relevant (Harding 2018). However, the reality of survival weakened the exceptionalism that many had previously attached to HIV (Rai, Bruton, Day, and Ward 2018). HIV-related death is now not inevitable, although mortality is still, unfortunately, higher among people with HIV compared with the general population (Croxford, Kitching, Desai et al. 2017). How to live, rather than how to die with HIV, has become the key narrative (Catalan, Ridge, Cheshire et al. 2020).

Coping with the shock and early horror of AIDS

An initial shock at the start of the epidemic was the dramatic rise in the cases of AIDS and the deaths associated with this increase. At this time, death was an inescapable reality for PLWH, their communities, and the NHS. Nevertheless, it is apparent that the intensity of the epidemic was at once traumatic and creative. As such, in the participants' narratives it can be seen that the long shadow of death not only traumatised people, but also energised them. Clearly, death continues to permeate modern-day narratives about HIV.

The experience of facing death and dying

It was not just the sheer number of deaths which was traumatising, but also the disturbing way in which many people tended to die. A gay man living with HIV described his feelings at the time and now:

> There were 12 of us on the ward, and in one week 8 died … in those days we were told to get ready to die, and we were dying, and dying in the most dreadful ways … it makes me so angry now, because people forget all those dying then.

Deaths were recalled as especially unpleasant, involving considerable pain, vomiting and diarrhoea, or breathing difficulties, among other distressing symptoms. The death of a partner could be particularly poignant, as in the case of this gay man living with HIV:

> I had seen death very close by the time my partner died. At Christmas, when he was allowed home, he wanted a bath in his own bathroom, and I could carry him up four flights of stairs in my arms, because he was about four stone. Is this what is going to happen to me? I had seen other people with monstrous carbuncles of KS on their face. I managed to hold everything together until after the funeral and then I completely went.

Unsurprisingly then, the emotions and trauma of this era were still present in our participants today, reverberating in the narratives we collected, and released by our questionings. The trauma was frequently expressed in emotional upset at the time of the interviews. A nurse described the personal toll of looking after dying people with HIV:

> When I went back to work on the ward I suddenly didn't know how to take blood pressure … I was getting terrible nightmares about the people who had died, and I had to stop for a while. I went back to it of course, but that was the time when I went, oh my

> *God, what the hell has just gone on there? It was like, I know people overuse the term, but it was like a war zone.*

Narratives from PLWH were infused with feelings of anger and shock, fear, and dread. There was a sense of decimation of entire friendship and support networks, including those of professionals. The empty address book became a familiar object of discussion. Summing up the losses, a physician recalled his experience:

> *This guy came in and handed me his address book and he had just crossed out the last name. He said, you might as well have it, because all his friends were gone.*

Nursing became an activity extending well beyond the immediate needs of patients, and it resulted in having to deal with death in all its intimate dimensions. A female nurse working in an HIV hospice described some of her duties:

> *We had a 12-bedded unit, and there would be people dying daily, and the nurses also managed the 12-bed mortuary. We would go to work and at the handover you would have a list of alive and dead patients, and for your shift you looked after both, and it meant going down to the mortuary and taking bodies out of the fridge and moving them to the viewing room.*

Considerable uncertainty about the best course of treatment, and its consequences, complicated matters. Treatment decisions were perceived as high stakes affairs, that could make the difference between life and death, such as in the case of failed treatment approaches which complicated matters and made choices very difficult, as recalled by a gay man living with HIV:

> *My partner decided to go on the AZT trial, while I decided I didn't want to take any pills, and within two years he started to fade as I got stronger from my cancer. He died in my arms later.*

For those working in HIV, many of whom came from the communities being devastated by the virus, grief and feelings of sadness had to be put to one side to deal with the unrelenting pressure to support and care for the sick. Clearly, looking after people with HIV on the wards and clinics in this pressurised environment took its toll on staff. Here, nursing staff constantly had to undertake work on the wards for which they had not been specifically trained, so they adapted their approaches as they went along:

> *As much as we tried to give people as good a death as possible, the deaths were often brutal … I had a guy come in and, I've never seen anybody so frightened in my life. He was absolutely terrified and he … there was such stigma, such a shame, and the press were awful. … and yeah so, this guy came in and he was really, really frightened, and he felt very humiliated because he couldn't walk. So he was having to crawl like a child on all fours and he looked at me and said, please, please, don't look at me like this … I am getting emotional, but I sat on the edge of his bed and he had his head on my chest,*

because I was trying to comfort him, stroking his hair, you wouldn't get away with it these days, but it was a beautiful moment actually. And yeah, he died and I was 21.

Medical and nursing staff, faced with no effective treatments, had to make an important shift in understanding their role, as a charity worker recalled:

Suddenly to have young people becoming very sick, very quickly, was a seismic shock, particularly to clinicians and nurses who had been trained to cure rather than primarily to care.

Doctors had to confront the reality of high death rates among their patients. Having been trained to diagnose and cure, they were unable to avoid the prospect of deterioration and death. A physician recalled the tasks he had to face:

You had to deal with the fact that people were going to die, you had to prepare them to die because they knew they would die … you didn't avoid talking about it.

The pressure of work and working conditions had an impact on medical staff, as described by this doctor in training at the time:

In that middle period, when it was very hectic, I mean, really, really, hectic, you got very tired. I routinely worked what wouldn't be allowed today, 80, 90, 100 hour weeks. Not because I was supposed to, but because I wanted to … and you get to the point when you think you are slightly invincible … and then occasionally it all breaks down, and I remember once sitting in an art gallery, and just crying.

These accounts of surviving PLWH, activists, nurses, doctors, and charity workers illustrate clearly the pain and despair experienced by those close to the continuous losses involved with the epidemic.

Responding to the experience of death

Faced with what seemed like an unstoppable flood of sickness and death, a wide range of responses occurred, sometimes leading to confronting death directly, and other times by attempting to change its meaning, or to avoid its impact by creating a distance from it.

Poignantly, the constant presence and trauma of death meant that living also became especially pressing and valued. Being forced to contemplate death led to positive changes, and to an increased focus on what really mattered to people at this stage in their lives. A charity worker described death as 'the magic ingredient' which resulted in people making changes to their lives in response to their increasing awareness of mortality:

I do think that the spectre of death was in a way the magic ingredient … we saw this extraordinary transformative process, people were having to face their own mortality and, in the process of doing it, they got good support and people were really figuring out in very new and different ways how to live.

Medical and nursing staff were also aware of the importance of those critical moments of end of life care, which in turn allowed them to deal with them in a reflective and positive manner. Within the wards, health professionals conveyed a sense of the privilege involved in working with people at the end of their lives, and were energised to continue caring and researching. A physician remembered such times:

> *It was an immense privilege to get to know those people towards the end of their lives, and it was a privilege to be part of what was a fantastic model of care … I think it gave our lives more meaning … and a huge understanding about what was precious about life, and it made it very special.*

It is not easy to appreciate how powerful the impact of looking after so many young people dying was at the time, when very little could be done to help, beyond attempting to minimise their suffering, as a physician recalled:

> *Yes, it was emotional, it hardened you, and it made many of us more adversarial for the fight, fighting to get drugs tested, evaluated with compassion and ethically … we took our strength from our early failures, from the deaths we remembered and the funerals we did or didn't go to.*

The positive personal consequences of dealing at this intense level of activity were tempered by their more obvious painful impact, both in the short and longer term. A female nurse working in a hospice reminisced about the pressures she and her colleagues experienced:

> *Working in the hospice was very formative in terms of self-awareness, about learning about yourself and about compassion and death and dying, and understanding that death is so part of life and that we live in such a death-denying culture and we are all so shocked when people die … but I guess you cannot live at that level of distress.*

For some, the consequences lived with them for a long time, never being entirely resolved, but also leading to positive moves. A charity worker recalled his own journey:

> *The death thing really gutted me and obviously changed me completely. I don't know what I would have been like if I hadn't been close to those things, and it makes me sad to think about it now … so yeah, when I reflect back on things like that it does make me, not depressed but intensely sad, but also it is bittersweet in a way … it did give me a thing to latch onto and work for and work towards.*

A change of role within the HIV service was an option for some, like this nurse, who found the experience overwhelming, and chose to move to a less exacting job, although still dealing with PLWH:

> *I did the outpatient clinic because I knew I couldn't do the wards anymore. I didn't admit it at the time, but I think there was something saying to me that it was, and of*

course nurses, we used to go to the patients' funerals as well. And at first, they were not fun, they were amazing things, but after a while you thought, I can't … I didn't have the emotional intelligence at 21 to deal with that.

Communication and mutual support were common within clinical teams, allowing informal access to sharing difficult feelings, often in preference to more formal supports. A psychiatric nurse recalled her experience of team support:

We talked to each other, we supported each other. The psychiatrist [in the team] was available but nobody went to see her … and only one person left, one of the consultants burnt out, he became unwell. But the rest of us stayed forever, working in one capacity or another, which is a measure of the way in which we did support each other.

Thus, individual efforts and team responses helped to set some limits on the experience, and to contain and manage some of the distress faced.

Funerals and other rituals

Funerals and their planning became an important feature of life on the hospital wards, and frequently became a creative response to the awful reality of sickness and death, even if that grim reality was sometimes quite stark. In the early days, families and friends only had a chance to say goodbye if they were present before or at the time when the person died, as remembered by a charity worker:

… and then there were the undertakers and the big, black, body bags … once dead, into the body bag … our charity had a list of good funeral directors and ones that were really difficult and really didn't want to deal with people with AIDS.

Participants recounted how funerals, or celebrations of life, were often planned in advance, with the dying person taking a direct role in organising the event. Friends and members of staff on the wards were frequently involved in this process, and in the subsequent funeral. A gay man living with HIV recalls the hospital ward atmosphere:

The wards were places of great contrast because you had mostly young men who were dying, but at the same time there was an element of laughter … we went to a lot of funerals, and they were such positive, colourful things, with show tunes instead of hymns … funerals became a celebration of life, not of sadness and loss.

Against all this sadness and trauma, creative responses followed, introducing a significant change in the way funerals were planned and organised. A charity worker remembered:

And very rapidly people wanted funerals to be celebrations of their life rather than solemn, the kind of funeral that you would have for your grandfather … there were some where their parents didn't want anyone to know, and the funeral would have eight or ten people, if that. On the other hand, there were those that were absolutely flamboyant and extraordinary, and with the coffin being brought in to "I will survive" by Gloria Gaynor, or a Pet Shop Boys track.

Confronting the approaching demise of the sick person and discussing death was not easy, but it helped people to gain some control over it, putting death in the wider context of the person's life. A psychiatrist remembered those difficult moments:

> *In those early days people would come with their living wills, and some funerals would be planned as well … I remember in one case the person choosing the music and who was to be invited, and he then jokingly asked for the video [of the funeral] to be sent to him … the way we dealt with the horror of it was by planning it and laughing, but it was still painful, we now think it was OK to talk about death in those days but it was still difficult, you had to face it, you couldn't pretend it wasn't going to happen.*

Preparing and attending funerals were not the only means for doctors and nurses to deal with death. Other rituals and routines were developed in some teams, for example, hospice rituals were recalled by a female nurse:

> *We used to have these sorts of routines, these rituals … whenever anybody died, we would open the window to let the spirit out and we would light a candle … it wasn't a religious thing, lots of people working there were atheists.*

Marking the passing of a person by acknowledging their presence and identity helped people involved in their care to get close to them before letting go. This experience of closeness and intimacy was described by a female HIV ward nurse:

> *In some cases, for some of those patients that I had laid out, that's a very intimate thing, like when you wash somebody for the final time and you do it with such respect of their dignity … the nurse who taught me how to lay somebody out who has died … she did it in such a way that was so humane and so respectful and so beautiful, that's a memory that I will hold forever. And I used to feel that that was my way of saying goodbye.*

Deciding whether to go to a funeral of a person the nurse or doctor had looked after sometimes required some reflection and balancing of outcomes. The dilemma faced by healthcare workers was recalled by a psychiatrist:

> *Should I go to my patients' funerals? Which funerals should I go to? Would it be a question of how involved I had been in the care of the person? Or of my previous contact with their family? I felt it would be too complicated for me to handle, apart from the question of personal as opposed to professional involvement, and maintaining some distance.*

Attempting to manage boundaries

The closeness between PLWH and nurses and doctors, and the intensity of the distress and emotion that characterised their contact, was not typical of the more traditional models of interaction between clinicians and patients in the average hospital ward or outpatient clinic. This was recognised by a PLWH:

> *The nursing staff and doctors, if they were able to, would come [to funerals] … the relationships, although sadly brief, were quite intense … we would all celebrate and mourn together … when you think about the level of loss that the people in the hospital had to deal with, the frustration, something that I think had almost been forgotten.*

For some clinicians, maintaining some distance was the way to protect their ability to cope and continue their task of caring for PLWH. A physician recalled:

> *As a doctor you cannot allow transference to occur, because otherwise you would never survive, but the difference from my perspective is that I had friends who were HIV positive, and three or four friends who had died, and I did find that extremely difficult at the time.*

Efforts to maintain the degree of emotional distance that would allow a doctor to continue functioning as a professional did not always work, as in the case of a paediatrician dealing with a very sick baby:

> *In fact, the first ever death we had of a little 3-month old baby with PCP, I looked after the baby, spoke to the parents and eventually we decided we would do nothing and the baby died. I did what I had to do, carried on, and the health visitor said, "I've never seen you cry, I didn't think you would." I think it is part of our training that you just cope with it … I did actually cry that time.*

As in the example above, the struggle to maintain some emotional distance could be difficult when faced with overwhelming human needs. Such struggles often took place in the absence of institutional support, as recalled by a ward nurse:

> *We were trained to cope, not to show emotion … if you said you wasn't coping well, it was as if you was a failure as a nurse … in those days there wasn't debriefing sessions, there wasn't any counselling, we just looked after each other. And of course, we were all going slightly bonkers in a way.*

In some hospital settings, awareness of professional boundaries was clearest among the mental health workers, who as a result of their training, were able to step back and assess the nature of the interaction with their patients, and the emotional demands that contact with sick and dying patients made on them. Frontline nurses and doctors were possibly less protected from the direct experience of serious illness and death, as a psychiatrist remembered:

> *I was struck by how involved with the patients the nurses in the medical team were, and how they would hug their patients or how they would go out drinking with them or*

> *even clubbing. There was a huge amount of personal involvement, and in our team, coming from mental health, we were much more aware of boundaries … I think [the nurses] felt we were uncaring because we kept a distance … rather than just jump in and hug patients, we would try to understand what was going on.*

The recognition of the consequences of having such fluid boundaries may have come too late for some of those involved in frontline work. The emotional impact of looking after very sick patients, although tempered by efforts to turn the pain into other emotions, like laughter – tears simultaneously of joy and sadness – was not entirely successful in terms of managing the boundaries, as some nurses reflected:

> *We needed to become more boundaried … I think, in hindsight, that it would have been better if we'd psychologically protected ourselves a little bit better.*

> *Then I started to get panic attacks and I didn't know why at the time … I was on the ward and suddenly I didn't know how to do a blood pressure, and I was getting terrible nightmares about people who had died … that KS was eating my lungs. I guess it was a form of post-traumatic stress … I never want to paint it out that it was all gloom, I've never laughed so much … the patients had me in tears, they were dying but they used to make me laugh because they were so funny.*

Some kind of progress

The slow Lazarus effect – are the graves empty now?

From the late 1980s onwards, some progress had taken place in the management of some of the manifestations of HIV. It is 1996, however, that is recognised as the year when significant changes to the treatment of HIV became realised. At the International AIDS Conference in Vancouver in 1996, the results of research showing the powerful effects of combination antiretroviral therapy (ART) were announced (Hammer et al. 1997), beginning a new chapter in the treatment of HIV infection.

Not everybody was convinced at the time about the long-term viability of ART, and there were concerns about a false dawn, given that there had been so many before. But as people started to take their new medication, many soon began to improve. This became known as the 'Lazarus effect', because improvements for some were dramatic, although for others it was a much more gradual improvement, as recalled by a heterosexual man living with HIV:

> *… the first and second drug combinations I went on didn't work, and it was the third one that very, very slowly started to help. They talked about the Lazarus effect, and it was Lazarus slowly.*

While the new treatments turned out to be the breakthrough everyone had been hoping for, the good news was often tainted by sadness and regret for those who had not survived long enough to receive them. Thus, in spite of the good news, people continued to die, and for some deaths were especially painful because of the increased hope surrounding them. Regrets at the missed opportunities and poor timing, continued over the years, and were particularly difficult because of the reminders of survival all around by then. A female community nurse recalled a poignant situation:

> *I remember one lady who is still around today, her baby was born with HIV and died when she was three months old, and it is still very raw for her, and very difficult for her to hear how well children are doing now.*

At this time of transition from despair to hope, the contrast between those who had missed their opportunity to have treatment in time and those who had received treatment and were improving, dampened the joy that should have come with greater survival, and contributed to some degree of survivors' guilt. Death continued to be associated with HIV, even if its significance was starting to shift. A charity worker remembered:

> *Post Vancouver it was great for some, but for others was too late, and that was, bittersweet doesn't begin to describe it, it was almost worse than before, because for those who it was too late for, they read all this good news, but it wasn't for them.*

Changes in services

Health care for PLWH began improving substantially in spite of initial doubts and uncertainties. Some of the services coping with high number of deaths started to become less relevant. Those workers whose lives had been dominated by HIV and its consequences, were able to start looking beyond it, and even think about a day when HIV ceased to be a problem, as recalled by a charity worker:

> *The really rapid drop in the number of funerals was such a relief … and it also allowed a lot of people who had been volunteering to leave and go off and do other things, to reacquaint themselves with their families or their gardens, or focus on gay adoption, for example.*

Specialised HIV hospices and wards, where sick and dying patients had been cared for, ceased to be an essential part of the system of care, and began to close or were amalgamated with other health areas. A female hospice nurse described some of the changes:

> *When the charity hospice started, the death rate was high, a lot of people chose to die there, but it finally closed … its garden is still there, it was a beautiful place that people loved … and one of the funny things was that there were lots of people's remains in the garden, lots of ashes, and the gardeners sent a memo asking people to stop scattering ashes because they were killing the plants. It was like there was too much blood and bone in the garden!*

New ethical dilemmas

The developing good news about survival also brought new ethical and practical decisions about when to treat actively, as opposed simply to try improving the person's quality of life, as this ward nurse explained:

> *We were beginning to get fewer patients on the ward ... and decisions about when to stop treatment became more difficult ... if we could begin to get people well permanently, then decisions about palliative care became much trickier. People didn't want to stop treating because there was a chance that they might survive.*

As the narratives quoted above show, the association of HIV with death had slowly and gradually started to loosen, with hope rising against a background of sadness and impotence.

'O death, where is thy sting?': living and dying with HIV now

> "It's bloody hard just staying alive ... I've been waiting to die for years," as one woman living with HIV recalled.

Once the immediate concerns about facing relentless death had receded, the focus shifted to planning a life with HIV, and not without complications. Current-day narratives in the field are predominantly focused not around death, but towards learning how to live and age well with the condition.

For many who had lived through the pre-ART era, learning to live in the shadow of death was a challenging prospect. They had not anticipated having a future. Many had been advised to spend their life savings while they could, and having not worked due to their illness had little savings or pension. With life-limiting disabilities and mental health problems, many had already mentally prepared for the prospect of an early death. A man with haemophilia recalled with wry humour:

> *The harder point for me, and I know for most haemophiliacs, was readjusting to: 'No, you are not going to get ill and die at some point ... you have to stop living like you are going to die soon, because you are not' ... Oh God, I've got to work for another 30 years, I was hoping to get ill, retire and die.*

HIV as a chronic illness, rather than a terminal condition, started to enter the HIV discourse, but the concept of 'chronic illness' when applied to HIV conceals complexity, in that individuals still struggle to survive, both in terms of their general health and ongoing mental difficulties, even if their struggles are less recognised in the prevailing discourse of a manageable condition. Even when physical heath is improved, exhaustion after many years of ill health and the aggregate experiences of loss, can make them an ill fit for the current healthcare paradigm. A gay man living with HIV summed up his predicament thus:

> *I have had HIV for 30 years, I have had a heart bypass, I am just finishing my third fight with cancer. I am used to learning how to survive ... my life's work these last 30 years has been surviving.*

The exhaustion resulting from many years of survival against the odds was described by a psychiatrist working with injecting drug users:

> *We have a cohort of people diagnosed for a long time who take their treatment well, but are exhausted by it, by the cumulative bereavements, by losing family and friends, and by feeling that the services around them have changed and probably do not meet their needs.*

Hope and joy are, however, certainly part of the work, as described by this nurse, who worked with women with HIV who became mothers in the current ART era:

> *[we worked] with many women and pregnancies, and babies born with HIV who died, generally. And then seeing these babies grow up, and in some cases our patients becoming grandparents … that was one of the joys of ART, that the women, once they were undetectable, could become pregnant again and the babies would not have HIV.*

Caring for people living with HIV now often became ordinary, almost mundane – who would have guessed? A charity worker reflected on the changes he had seen from the start of the epidemic to the present time:

> *It is nice to reflect back and think, oh God, it was so awful then and there was nothing we could do … so to have it as it is now, to have it so normalised so people think it is over, is I guess kind of funny, but it is almost good in the sense that it is boring, it's not in the news because no one's dying, obviously there's still needs but because it is not in the news, that's great.*

Denial of death becomes possible again

A number of participants were concerned that effective HIV treatment had allowed a death-denying culture to return. There was some unease that with death now being less likely, and 'the magic ingredient' being lost, the refocusing of attention on living well, had been lost also. The 'death literacy' (Spence 1996) that had been acquired in the early days, which included the ability to talk about and confront death more openly, was thought to have receded: death could again be seen as a kind of failure. Health professionals, like this doctor, described how current HIV deaths could be more difficult to deal with, and seen as a failure, due to their perceived preventability:

> *People with HIV still die, and it is harder for medics now, knowing that the expectation is that HIV is treatable, and that death is not meant to happen.*

Medical staff can be caught up in the denial or avoidance of the death topic, as recalled by a psychiatrist:

> *Sometimes treatment doesn't work, even after trying different medications, and it becomes very difficult for the medics, because they sense that – I can't save you, it shouldn't*

happen. It is hard for them to deal with this, hence the problem of dealing with death now, when it shouldn't happen, and it becomes something secretive, something not to be talked about.

For those diagnosed in the current ART era, death although very much part of the collective HIV consciousness, is often not something that PLWH need to think about in conjunction with their diagnosis. A gay man living with HIV gave this straightforward response:

I guess death is something I never think about, it is just a case of a) die, or b) take your medication and live. It is a very simple choice.

All of which led a charity worker to sum up the current situation:

Recent changes have perhaps enabled our death-denying culture to creep back.

Memories of death and loss are still around us

Despite death being less frequently discussed, the legacy of the early crisis of inevitable deaths, and the spectre of trauma surrounding those deaths still permeates the current narratives. For PLWH the sense of decimation of friendship networks frequently led to social isolation, adding to the difficulties of adjusting to long-term survival in a changed world. PLWH were also left with the memories of the pre-ART era, including the friends they lost, not to mention the loss of their own youth to HIV, as recalled by these gay men living with HIV:

I lost my peer group, really, and they haven't been replaced … it would have been nice to have those people with us still.

People post pictures of friends [who have died] on Facebook and I just cannot bear to look … I just prefer to have it locked away in a sense.

For PLWH, talking during therapy or in discussions with close friends allowed some reflections on what they had faced, their own mortality, and contemporary issues of dying, such as those related to recreational drug-taking:

We have regular conversations now, and it is about so-and-so has died, and it's either heart attack, suicide, but at the core of both of those is drugs.

Some described their lack of tolerance for those newly diagnosed who had not lived through the 'war', as they well remembered the trauma of the pre-ART years. A physician remembered:

My willingness to put up with people saying 'Oh, I can't take this pill once a day it's too big' or 'I can't swallow pills', it's like, well fuck off and die then … you've caught an infection, you are going to have to take pills for the rest of your life. Take your pill, and then come back and see me in six months, bugger off.

For many the startling reversal in their plight was highlighted by realising that it was their doctors and nurses, who had looked after them for many years, who were now retiring or dying. These were the health professionals who had looked after PLWH for decades. Professional careers were initially set to outlive PLWH by some considerable time, and now it is the long-standing patients who are being abandoned. A ward nurse recalled with some sadness:

> *Patients talk about their doctors, whom they have been seeing for years, and now the doctors are ageing and retiring, and they never thought they would see their doctors retire … we were telling them that they were going to leave us, and in fact, we are leaving them. They do feel a sense of loss and bereavement.*

The new deaths in PLWH

As a ward nurse regretfully said:

> *So, I'd get patients coming in going, oh well, I don't want to take these drugs because I take E on Fridays – and in my head I'd be going, people would have gone over broken glass to get these drugs. Drugs, chemsex, that's fuelling a lot of HIV now, and is having a devastating effect on people!*

Despite now having reached a historical high point in HIV treatment, there are still ongoing challenges faced by many populations at risk of HIV which lead to premature death. This is the sting in the tail of the Lazarus effect. At the heart of these are ongoing mental health problems and stigma. Recreational drug using among men who have sex with men (MSM) and other groups can become chaotic, presenting mental health challenges, not to mention those of adhering to life-saving HIV medication regimens. In the UK, for MSM the chemsex scene in particular has grown in recent years, leaving many men addicted and vulnerable. The irony of living through the HIV crisis to witness modern chemsex deaths was not lost on this ward nurse:

> *It's changed and there is still the psychological stuff, but of course the big thing now is chemsex. Now we are seeing people die of drugs, which is really hard for me to see. We've had four deaths from G[HB] this year. I cannot see another group of young men die.*

For African immigrants on the other hand, stigma is still so high that diagnosis and treatment can be dangerously compromised, and there is concern that many still die shortly after diagnosis (Pantazis, Thomadakis, del Amo et al. 2019).

The legacy and further challenges

As our participants illustrate, there has been a significant change in the narratives about HIV death and dying, from the terrible pain of loss and anger of the early days, to the hesitant expectation of change, and finally the acceptance of hope. Death generated creative and empowering responses which influenced not just PLWH but also their voluntary and professional carers.

Believing in hope: things can change

We have witnessed the change within a generation, from the devastation of the early years to the controlled and largely successful treatment of PLWH who have access to ART. A new and deadly disease has been understood, and effective treatment strategies developed. At the same time, the associated stigma and its wider social impact are being tackled. If the evidence from Switzerland is in any way applicable to the UK, mortality from suicide among PLWH will have declined substantially in the last three decades (Ruffieux, Lemsalu, Aebi-Popp et al. 2019), further contributing to the drop in HIV-related deaths.

We discuss below how some of the lessons from the past are at risk of being forgotten, as the memories of shock and death fade, and newly diagnosed PLWH and their doctors and nurses live in a milieu far less dramatic. A nurse who had been on the frontline of caring for PLWH for many years reflected on the change:

> *I remember how powerful that time was, the impact it had on us … when I was younger, I used to listen to war veterans, and I used to think, oh for god's sake … I get them now.*

The major shift in the way the narratives of death and dying with HIV have changed over four decades provides a model for successful intervention for other seemingly intractable health problems. The collaborative work of the affected communities, together with the efforts of scientists, clinicians, and politicians, show the way forward.

Learning to talk about death and the risk of losing this skill

As the widespread use of effective antiretroviral treatment improved the prognosis of PLWH, a sense of hope and relief started to emerge. As discussed elsewhere (Catalan et al. 2020), responses to these changes have not always been predictable. For example, Rofes (1998) argued strongly for a post-AIDS perspective, writing about "stuffing the red ribbon rhetoric" and "the Quilt having outlived its purpose", and "leaving aside the funereal feelings". There is some concern, however, that an understandable consequence of the undeniable progress we have experienced has been the loss of death literacy and the return of a death-denying culture.

Outside the context of HIV, there has been a growing literature discussing death in medical settings, mostly written by doctors exposed to death on a daily basis. This literature highlights the limits of medical intervention in the context of dealing with progressive conditions and terminal care, and how the complexity of choices and treatments available can distract from the facts at hand (Gawande 2014; O'Mahony 2016). As in the days of high mortality in PLWH, those closely involved in dealing with death in medical settings recognise the desirability of talking about death and naming it, confronting the fears associated with it, and planning ahead (Mannix 2017).

It could be argued with Rofes that living with HIV, rather than obsessing about death, is the right approach when the individual is in good health, a period which may well last many years. The problem, however, is about bringing back death literacy, especially when a PLWH develops serious complications and has to consider the reality of an approaching end. The loss of death literacy may make it harder for the individual to make a realistic appraisal now, perhaps falling back on the 'fighting talk' and 'battling the disease' clichés that can prevent people from discussing end of life wishes (Macmillan Cancer Support 2018). Integrating palliative care into the overall care of people with HIV has been shown to be effective in enhancing patient-centred care, affirming life and regarding dying as a normal process (Harding 2018). Contrary to received wisdom, rather than becoming less important over time, death in HIV has morphed into different forms and guises. Instead of being seen as a marker of failure and decay, we argue it has never been a more essential consideration for living and dying well.

Funerals as celebrations of life

It is not uncommon nowadays for funerals to be not just a time for mourning, but also celebrations of people's lives. In what is claimed to be the largest study of funeral customs in the UK by a funeral care organisation (Co-operative Funeral Care 2011, 2019), the increase of non-traditional ceremonies and the range of options available for music and words, dress, and flowers or donations, among others, illustrates how in recent years there has been a significant change in the way the final goodbye is organised. Funeral historians and researchers stress that individualised and personal funeral rituals have always existed (Field, Hockey, and Small 1997), although it is only in recent years that they have started to replace traditional religious funerals (Litten 2002).

Funerals of people dying from HIV, sometimes with striking and colourful expressions of grief and celebration, evoked intense feelings in individuals and communities that helped them to cope, while also making statements of resilience and strength by and for those frequently perceived as living outside traditional social norms. While it is not possible to prove conclusively that AIDS funerals were the main factor in the increased popularity of non-traditional funerals in general, it is quite likely that they contributed to this public shift, perhaps pushing against a half-open door. A charity worker speculated about the ripple effect of funerals of people dying with HIV in a wider context:

> *HIV funerals did have an impact, because some of them were broadcast as part of real life documentaries of the lives of people with AIDS, and with such a large number of deaths, many people went to funerals one way or another … funerals don't need to be the way they were in the past, music is chosen, and they are much more like a celebration, rather than just grief and loss, but without losing the importance of the funeral to say goodbye.*

Self-protection and managing boundaries

Participants, especially those involved in frontline care and support of people dying with HIV, often talked about the tension between wanting a close intimacy with their patients and the pain and sadness resulting from the subsequent losses. A sense of privilege and purpose and personal growth was tempered for some by enduring sadness, post-traumatic stress disorder, and long-term depression (Cheshire, Ridge, Hedge et al. 2019). A physician with many years' experience of dedicated work, described his exhaustion and eventual retirement:

> *I started to lose empathy … this is the point at which I don't think I can do this anymore … maybe the younger people can do it because they haven't seen all the death. They don't have the legacy behind them weighing them down, and there is a time to leave.*

Many health professionals could distance themselves by using their scientific work as a way of coping, and others diversified their work by transferring to less demanding tasks, away from direct contact with patients, or simply by leaving their position. Informal support within cohesive teams as well as support groups that met regularly or as needed were alternative ways to maintain some perspective. As in the example given above, specific therapy was sometimes required (Bayer and Oppenheimer 2000, p207–214).

Making a decision of whether or not to attend funerals and in what circumstances to do so, is another example of how people dealt with boundaries between their professional and personal roles. US physicians in the early days of the epidemic described a range of responses to the question of funerals, from those who had decided early on they would not attend, to those who were selective on the basis of previous involvement with the deceased and their families, and those who found it logistically impossible to attend so many funerals. A self-protective element was present in many such instances (Bayer and Oppenheimer 2000, p203–207), something that rings true in the UK too. There is no easy solution to these questions, which are nowadays discussed more widely, beyond HIV care (McCartney 2018).

The return of the repressed: memories and echoes

In spite of Rofes' optimism, for the generation that has lived through the epidemic, early losses remain a persistent and emotionally laden memories, summed up by Augustine of Hippo as 'The dead are invisible, they are not absent'. Death thus never ends, it only transforms, e.g. into the ageing and dying of the first HIV care professionals, and the death of gay men from drug use and mental health-related problems, or of Black African people from a delayed diagnosis. We have to face the less conscious concerns around HIV and death, even among those that have a hopeful, optimistic view of their clinical prognosis. In the case of gay men in particular, there remains a culture of shame, difficulties with self-acceptance, and seeking refuge in strategies for short-term escape from uncomfortable feelings, such as recreational drug use, alcohol misuse, or sex (Catalan et al. 2020). Denial of death in this context may be another way of avoiding difficult feelings linked to the long-term shadow cast by HIV infection, not to mention homophobia itself, which linked gayness to death and destruction long before HIV came along (Downs 2005; Todd 2018).

Conclusions

The narratives about death and HIV have changed significantly over the years, from the overwhelming sadness and trauma of the early days, through to the development of a 'death literacy' that improved the care of PLWH, and led to creative responses. While now PLWH, activists, and health and charity workers have begun to distance themselves from those early experiences, many still live under the long shadow of death. Its denial has become possible, and it may even be seen as a failure now that there are effective treatments.

Death also reverberates in the choice to live better and find ways to care for PLWH, something that a number of people touched by the early epidemic discussed. The early years of dealing with HIV forced those involved in the struggle to face what was perceived as inevitable death to develop ways of confronting and transcending it, a pioneering movement that subsequent progress in the treatment of HIV has weakened. It is understandable that the sense of hope and survival associated with HIV infection today would lead to forgetting in the UK poor outcomes and the lessons from the past.

References

Bayer R and Oppenheimer GM (2000) *AIDS doctors: voices from the epidemic*. Oxford, Oxford University Press.

Blair C and Michel N (2007) The AIDS memorial quilt and the contemporary culture of public commemoration. *Rhetoric and Public Affairs*, 10(4): 595–626.

Cantacuzino M (1993) *Till break of day*. London, William Heinemann Ltd.

Catalan J, Ridge D, Cheshire A, Hedge B, and Rosenfeld D (2020) The changing narratives of death, dying, and HIV in the UK. *Qualitative Health Research*, 30(10): 1561–1571. doi:10.1177/1049732320922510

Cheshire A, Ridge D, Hedge B, and Catalan J (2019) "It's all marvelous now on the face of it, but there is a lot of hurt": narratives of those working on the frontline. *AIDS IMPACT 14th International Conference*, London, Session 59.

Co-operative Funeral Care (2011) *The ways we say goodbye*, www.heartofenglandfuneralcare.co.uk

Co-operative Funeral Care (2019) *Burying traditions: the changing face of UK Funerals*, www.heartofenglandfuneralcare.co.uk

Croxford S, Kitching A, Desai S, Kall M, Edelstein M, Skingsley A, Burns F, Copas A, Brown A, Sullivan A, and Delpech V (2017) Mortality and causes of death in people diagnosed with HIV in the era of highly active antiretroviral therapy: an analysis of a national observational cohort. *Lancet Public Heath*, 2(1): e35–e46.

Downs A (2005) *The velvet rage*. Philadelphia, PA, Da Capo Press, Perseus Book Group.

Field D, Hockey J, and Small N (ed) (1997) *Death, gender and ethnicity*. London, Routledge.

Garfield S (1994) *The end of innocence*. London, Faber & Faber.

Gawande A (2014) *Being mortal*. London, Profile Books.

Hammer SM, Squires KE, Hughes MD, Grimes JM, Demeter LM, Currier JS, Eron JJ, Feinberg JE, Balfour HH, Deyton LR, Chodakewitz JA, and Fischl MA (1997) A controlled trial of two nucleoside analogues plus indinavir in persons with HIV infection. AIDS Clinical Trials Group 320 Study Team. *New England Journal of Medicine*, 337(11): 725–733.

Harding R (2018) Palliative care as an essential component of the HIV care continuum. *The Lancet*, 5(10): E524–E530. doi:10.1016/52352-3018(18)30110-3

King M (2013) How The Denver Principles changed healthcare forever. *POZ*, 7 June, https://www.poz.com/blog/how-the-denver-princ

Litten J (2002) *The English way of death: the common funeral since 1450*. London, Robert Hale & Company.

Macmillan Cancer Support (2018) *Missed oppportunities: advance care planning report*, www.macmillan.org.uk

Mannix K (2017) *With the end in mind: dying, death, and wisdom in an age of denial*. London, HarperCollins.

McCartney M (2018) Should doctors go to patients' funerals? *British Medical Journal*, 362: 21; 362:sek2865.

Morolake O, Stephens D, and Welbourn J (2009) Greater involvement of people living with HIV in health care. *Journal of the International AIDS Society*, 12(1):4. doi:10.1186/1758-2652-12-4

Nuland SB (1994) *How we die*. London, Chatto & Windus Ltd.

O'Mahony S (2016) *The way we die now*. London, Head of Zeus Ltd.

Pantazis N, Thomadakis C, del Amo J, Alvarez-del Arco D, Burns F, Fakoya I, and Toulumi G (2019) Determining the likely place of HIV acquisition for migrants in Europe combining subject-specific information and biomarkers data. *Statistical Methods in Medical Research*, 28(7): 1979–1997. doi:10.1177/096220217746437

Rai T, Bruton J, Day S, and Ward H (2018) From activism to secrecy: contemporary experiences of living with HIV in London in people diagnosed from 1986 to 2014. *Health Expectations*, 21(8): 108. doi:10.1111/hex.12816

Rofes E (1998) *Dry bones breathe: gay men creating post-AIDS identities and cultures*. New York, Harrington Park Press.

Rosenfeld D, Bartlam B, and Smith RD (2012) Out of the closet and into the trenches: gay male baby boomers, ageing, and HIV/AIDS. *The Gerontologist*, 52(2): 255–264.

Ruffieux Y, Lemsalu L, Aebi-Popp K, Calmy A, for the Swiss HIV Cohort Study and the Swiss National Cohort (2019) Mortality from suicide among people living with HIV and the general Swiss population: 1988–2017. *Journal of the International AIDS Society*, 22: e25339.

Shilts R (1987) *And the band played on*. London, Penguin Books.

Spence C (1996) *On watch*. London, Cassell.

Todd, M (2018) *Straight jacket: overcoming society's legacy of gay shame*. London, Black Swan, Penguin Random House.

8 Changing attitudes to sexuality and HIV

Introduction

Prior to the start of the HIV epidemic in the USA and UK, there had been important moves in the direction of fighting for the rights of lesbians, gay men, trans, and queer people (LGBTQ). The 1969 New York Stonewall Inn riots in response to ongoing police harassment of LGBTQ patrons, although not the first, represent a watershed moment that had symbolic meaning as marking the start of gay liberation (Armstrong and Crage 2006). Gay liberation joined other liberation movements, such as those for the rights of Blacks in the US and feminist movements worldwide, to demand society change. Major challenges to the inferior roles assigned to women in society took place in the aftermath of the two World Wars, when women had been able to take on traditional male jobs in the absence of men. Additionally, with the increasing availability later of the oral contraceptive pill, female sexuality was gradually untied from child rearing. However, disapproving attitudes to same-sex behaviours remained.

The start of the HIV epidemic in the early 1980s was a challenge to progressive developments, when sexual liberation in general – and homosexuality in particular – were portrayed by the political powers and the media at the time as having led to a major health crisis. Worse still, for conservative commentators, the survival of the family and society were considered at risk from homosexuality. With the US President Ronald Reagan and the UK Prime Minister Margaret Thatcher in power, a conservative and neoliberal world was taking shape in western democracies, and social attitudes against homosexual behaviour hardened. These were the years when the impact of HIV infection was at its most devastating, with increasing rates of infection and mortality, accompanied by prominently negative and sensationalist media reporting.

Four decades later, and the landscape is considerably different, at least in much of the so-called developed world. Social attitudes have changed significantly in the direction of a more positive attitude towards male and female same-sex relationships, despite recent negative developments, such as open hostility to trans people – especially trans women – by a section of UK feminists (Hines 2019). Legislative protections regarding same-sex sexual behaviour and relationships in a wide range of areas, from age of consent, to civil partnership and same-sex marriage, adoption, human fertilisation, antidiscrimination legislation, amongst others, have been established in the UK.

How has this happened? What led to such significant shifts in public attitudes and progressive legislation, at a time when the HIV epidemic and its impact were perceived in such negative terms? Did HIV itself play a part in bringing about these changes?

Here we argue how the early role of HIV community organisations and activism in alerting both the public, and government and public health officials, together with the action of committed health workers and progressive politicians and civil servants, brought into the open topics hitherto avoided in public discourse. These included same-sex sexual practices and relationships, and sexually explicit HIV prevention campaigns. More open discussions led to a greater visibility of minority groups, a gradual liberalisation in discourses, and a reappraisal of same-sex behaviour and relationships. However, as recent political history shows, progressive changes once established are not secured once and for all, and must be continually fought for.

The 1950s and 1960s – a time of change

It was not until the after the Second World War that laws against sexual activity between males that were first enacted more than 400 years earlier and modified subsequently, started to be revoked. King Henry VIII's Buggery Act of 1533, repealed by Queen Mary in 1553 but re-enacted by Elizabeth I 10 years later, punished buggery with death, while the Offences against the Person Act 1861 reduced this to life imprisonment. The Criminal Law Amendment Act 1885, the Labouchere Amendment, extended laws about homosexuality to include any sexual activity between males. Oscar Wilde was convicted under this Act in 1895.

Reform movements in the late 1890s and early 1900s, in what Weeks (2016, p115–126) has described as "the creation of a consciousness", began a new and uncertain process, against a background of repression and prosecutions. The trial in 1954 of three socially prominent men – Lord Montague; Peter Wildeblood, a journalist; and Michael Pitt-Rivers, a landowner – for committing acts of "conspiracy to incite male persons to commit serious offences with male persons", led to public debate about the law regarding homosexual offences, and resulted in the setting up of a committee to review it. The Wolfenden Report, as the 1957 committee's report was called, recommended that homosexual behaviour between consenting adults in private should no longer be a criminal offence.

The fact that it took another 10 years before the Sexual Offences Act 1967 (England and Wales) was passed, reflects the degree of debate and controversy involved. This limited decriminalisation of homosexual acts only applied to men over 21 years old, and the acts had to be in private (Weeks 2016, p155–181). Thus, theoretically, if the sexual act took place in a hotel room or in any place where others were present, it could be interpreted as occurring in public, and therefore illegal.

Discussions became prominent in the context of heterosexual relationships, with perceptions of love, courtship, and marriage becoming more fluid, and undergoing significant changes from the mid-century years onwards (Langhamer 2013). For instance, the contraceptive pill became available on the NHS in 1961, although initially only to married couples. This medical development gave women, in particular, the ability to separate sexual activity from procreation, helping to usher in the so-called 'sexual revolution'. This was a time of broader social change and unrest, with Black liberation movements in the US, the 1968 students' and workers' industrial action in France, the Prague spring, and the anti-Vietnam war demonstrations in the US.

Many gay organisations had been formed by 1969 in the US in support of the rights of homosexuals, and the police raid of the New York gay bar, the Stonewall Inn, in June of the same year led to rioting that proved a highly symbolic turning point – no longer would LGBTQ people put up with harassment from the authorities. What's more, rights were being demanded. The New York Gay Liberation Front arose from the Stonewall revolt, and it was followed on this side of the Atlantic with the foundation in 1970 of the London Gay Liberation Front (GLF). Gay Pride marches began in 1971, and London GLF had links with other movements fighting the oppression of women, workers, and the policies of the Conservative government of Edward Heath (1970–1974) (Weeks 2016, p185–206). While GLF later seemed to lose focus, it initiated a period of development and growth of organisations such as the Campaign for Homosexual Equality (CHE) in 1971, Friend in 1975, and the newspaper *Gay News* in 1972, contributing to the development of gay communities centred mostly in major inner city areas (Weeks 2016, p207–230).

In spite of these changes and undeniable progress, legal discrimination and negative attitudes continued, and difficulties coming out to parents, work colleagues, and employers, were considerable. Public attitudes towards homosexuality were mixed and somewhat alarming. The British Social Attitudes Survey reported that between 1979 and 1981, 62% of people favoured legalisation of homosexual relations. Yet even in 1983, when the AIDS panic started, 62% thought that homosexual acts were "always or mostly wrong" (Jowell, Whitherspoon, and Brook 1988, p111 and p125), suggesting that while legal changes and greater visibility of the gay community and gay and lesbian organisations had led to some grudging acceptance amongst the general population, disapproval was still prevalent.

The 1980s: the HIV epidemic puts the brakes on progress, and yet…

As the AIDS epidemic emerged in the 1980s, and within the next few years as the epidemic unfolded, some of the activists who had been involved in struggles to support gay people and advance their rights became those who set up charities and organisations to educate gay people who were at risk of becoming infected with HIV. They took an active role in counteracting the negative publicity and stigmatisation against AIDS that the mainstream media encouraged, exploiting the negative public attitudes to homosexuality prevalent in the previous decades.

Not surprisingly, however, obtaining funding for these organisations was often difficult, as described by one charity worker:

> At first there was no public funding for charities, and when we tried to get funding from
> the local council for personnel, another council took them to court to prevent the grant being

> paid. *The environment at the time was such that when the London Lesbian and Gay Switchboard had applied in 1981 to the Charity Commission for charitable status, they were refused on the basis that providing information and support to homosexuals was not a proper charitable activity. We learnt from that, and so when we applied for charitable status in 1984, we did so as an AIDS organisation, which was enormously helpful.*

The conservative political context was relevant: Margaret Thatcher was elected Prime Minister in 1979, followed by subsequent victories in 1983 and 1987. A strong conservative agenda, both socially and economically, with a clear neoliberal approach, became dominant. As stated by Weeks, "enduring efforts to separate the 'implicated' from the 'immune', the 'guilty' from the 'innocent', spoke to a culture which feared the impact of sexual change, social complexity, and moral diversity" (Weeks 1995, p16). The UK government initially distanced itself from the impending crisis, unsure as to how to respond, and no significant government response took place until 1986 (Weeks 2007, p17).

First steps: activists, public health officials, and government ministers

The Chief Medical Officer, Sir Donald Acheson, who regarded AIDS as a public health problem, rather than a moral one, began in late 1984 to discuss the developing situation with gay activists. The testimonies of gay activists from the coalface illustrate the emergent contacts between the official responsible for public health and the community groups most affected by AIDS.

> *It started, very early on in 1985, with my hearing that the Department of Health was thinking of a public health education campaign around AIDS. So, I thought that maybe somebody who had HIV could offer some advice about it and have a perspective on what it might be that the government might say. So, I wrote to the Department of Health saying exactly that, and there was a phone call from the Department of Health saying that the Chief Medical Officer would like to meet you … it led to the formation of the first advisory committee on public education, and it was to this group that the Department brought its proposals about the first advertising campaign.*

> *We rapidly had meetings with the Chief Medical Officer, Sir Donald Acheson, and I remember he actually phoned us and said he wanted to talk. Which was brilliant, and then with government ministers, and going up from juniors to cabinet level … there was a recognition that this was a health crisis that needed to be handled sensitively.*

> *Sir Donald Acheson, CMO, gave us his home number and said call me after 7 o'clock because then there won't be any civil servants around, and because he, as an epidemiologist, understood how epidemics worked, and he knew that a community action to prevent its spread could only be delivered by gay men, a huge, a real foresight.*

The public health versus morality debate reached the highest levels of government. Margaret Thatcher's reservations about paying attention to AIDS extended to her efforts to stop government-funded research into sexual behaviours across the UK population that could help assess and predict the current and future patterns of

HIV spread. As described by Wellings et al. (1994, p8–12), carefully planned research by epidemiologists and statisticians already approved in 1987 by the Department of Health and ready to start field work in 1989, was then "put on ice without explanation". According to press reports this was as a result of Downing Street claiming it would be an invasion of privacy and an inappropriate use of public funds (Wellings et al. 1994, p11). Fortunately, the Wellcome Trust stepped in and provided the funds for research plans to be resumed. The National Survey of Sexual Attitudes and Lifestyles was born, and has so far led to three major sets of data gathered in 1990, 1999, and 2010 (Wellings et al. 1994; Johnson, Wadsworth, Wellings, and Field 1994; Johnson, Mercer, Erens, Copas et al. 2001; Mercer, Tanton, Prah, Erens et al. 2013).

It is interesting to note that similar debates were taking place in the USA. The Reagan administration had tried to avoid facing up to the HIV crisis, and it was the Surgeon General, Dr C Everett Koop, a born-again Christian, who against much political conservative pressure launched a publicity campaign in 1988, sending an educational brochure to every household in the US (France 2016, p317). As in the UK, the adoption of a public health message rather than moralising about sexual behaviours or denying reality, proved to be shrewd.

Crucial to the development of a strategy to deal with the impending AIDS epidemic was the recognition in the mid-1980s by public health officials and government ministers of the need to work together with gay community organisations and with doctors to tackle a major health crisis. A charity worker remembered those early days:

> There was no history in 1984 of either the government or civil service working with lesbians and gay men, nor was there any expertise, or very limited, amongst gay men about how to go about talking to government. At that time, at the height of the Thatcher government there was real reluctance for the civil service to allow ministers to be seen to be influenced by 'gay radicals', because at that time, if you were a lesbian or gay man, or working or volunteering for THT or the London Lesbian and Gay Switchboard, you were by definition a radical left winger.

The debates about morality continued, however, and the anti-permissive crusade of the third Thatcher government was illustrated by the Prime Minister's address to the Conservative party conference in 1987. Here she told delegates that "children who need to be taught to respect traditional moral values are being taught that they have an inalienable right to be gay" (Watney 1989, p23; Cook 2017a, p58). Most notorious was the passing of Clause 28 of the Local Government Act of 1988, later known as Section 28, which banned "the intentional promotion of homosexuality" by local authorities and "teaching the acceptability of homosexuality as a pretended family relationship". Paradoxically, it had the opposite effect by becoming a focal point of a growing mobilisation to dismantle the legislation, both by gay and lesbian community groups, as well as by the more progressive sections of society, thus increasing the visibility of gays and lesbians (Watney 1989, p21–26; Weeks 2016, p242–244; Cook 2017a, p58–59; Cook 2017b, p251–258). Section 28 was finally repealed by the Labour government in 2003 in the face of fierce opposition from the Conservatives and their supporters.

A nurse who had been on the front line of caring for people living and dying with HIV explained how Section 28 struck a nerve, harnessing the anger of activists:

> *In the middle of this, Clause 28 came out, and that was a fucking cruel thing to bring out at the time. We had lots of people against us, it was very political, but you had a group of people who were losing their lovers and friends, and they weren't going to take it anymore. And thank God for them activists, they got the drugs out, Pride became political, we used to take patients in wheelchairs to Pride … it is not politicians that change things, it is people that change things, this was a prime example, it was phenomenal.*

Activists, the media, and Princess Diana

The popular media played an important part in highlighting public concerns, but not usually in an accurate, impartial way. Even the more responsible and thoughtful media outlets were often caught up in an atmosphere of sensationalism (Alcorn 1989, p193–212). Nevertheless, aspects of media debates were perceived as ultimately positive by many, like this gay man living with HIV:

> *There was a lot of media in the early days … sometimes they could be incredibly helpful in creating an environment where people realised we were making progress, and I think it influenced politicians because they realised that putting money into the NHS that could offer world-class care would be cost effective.*

A particularly significant event that the media highlighted and which had an impact on the public perception of people living with HIV (PLWH), was the visit on 19 April 1987 of Princess Diana to the London's Middlesex Hospital, to open a ward specifically designed to treat people with HIV. Princess Diana was photographed sitting and shaking hands without wearing gloves with a person with AIDS. It has been claimed since then that this gesture, repeated in future occasions when she visited hospitals and hospices, played a critical role in reducing stigma and increasing the acceptance of PLWH. Views about Princess Diana are now more nuanced than they were at the time, with criticism of her use of the media and her personal limitations, together with praise for her support of worthy causes. The comments of a nurse and a doctor reported here acknowledge her positive role in relation to AIDS:

> *Princess Diana changed the face of HIV. I'm not a royalist, but that woman had a big heart. She made a difference to HIV.*

> *I think science made a commitment because it was a real, public health risk … I think the UK government responded extremely well. People like Norman Fowler, and no matter what you might think of Princess Diana, she was a really important part.*

Activists were also able to use the media to highlight the plight of gay people and to raise funds for HIV charities, often involving celebrities and other influential individuals, in an attempt to alter negative perceptions about HIV. An activist and charity worker recalled those days:

> We did a lot of TV and radio work, and we had really moving letters and phone calls saying you have given me courage to tell my parents that I'm gay … fund raising with people like Stephen Fry, Simon Callow, Elton John, and George Michael, and knowing that we were having an impact … there were only four TV channels at the time, and so if you were on the 9 or 10 o'clock news, you knew that most people in the country had seen it one way or another.

The media exposure of activists and their messages had the effect of moving the focus of discussion away from generalised views about 'AIDS victims' or socially unacceptable 'risk groups' towards the acceptance of PLWH as articulate and committed individuals, who were able to make a rational and compassionate case about the need for action. As a charity worker stated:

> What the LGBT community was doing in response to a national, global crisis gave us faces, and stressed the importance of telling people stories in the media about HIV, and the same for a move towards gay equality.

The formation of alliances continues

Behind the scenes, the contacts initiated in the early 1980s between public health officials and activists continued and rapidly led to the inclusion of PLWH and other activists on government advisory committees and local authority panels. Coalition building with local authorities, politicians, and health officials, as well as doctors and their professional organisations, became a necessary development. This sometimes slow but continuous growth in contacts between activists, public health officials, medical organisations and individual doctors, and PLWH, contributed to a shift in attitudes amongst influential bodies and individuals, and added to the pressures for a change in social attitudes. An activist and charity worker remembered the importance of creating alliances:

> By this point it was clear that gay men on their own could never deal with it, so we had to make alliances, and any of our friends were more than welcome, so the number of women involved as volunteers continued to grow. By 1985 there was a medical group, a health promotion group, 'buddy' group, helpline group, social services group to work with directors of social services.

Political contacts were not limited to conversations between activists, government ministers and officials. Activists also reached towards other political parties, planting the seeds of change amongst opposition politicians, as this charity worker remembered:

> The charity was at all political party conferences from 1989, and it was those meetings that brought people like Tony Blair into discussion and dialogue.

Alliances continued to be formed, in this instance between PLWH, activists, and doctors and researchers, all parties recognising the value of this new form of coalition building. A long-standing physician recalled the novelty and range of the involvement of people with HIV with doctors and others:

> *I don't think I had ever experienced patient groups in this way, obviously there had been things like the Patients Association and things like that. This was a very much more political, thrusting sort of thing, trying to get HIV on the political agenda.*

The involvement of PLWH in campaigning, research, and practical organisation of services in collaboration with their doctors became the common pattern, as remembered by a senior physician:

> *I think that one of the great things with HIV is the way in which the patient groups sorted themselves out, insisted on better food, insisted on liberal laws, so they often went into serious advocacy, insisted on the best randomised trial as quickly as possible … I think patient activism was a source of great good … most activism was unbelievably helpful.*

However, the cross currents of conservatism and progressive forces seemed to clash at this historical point, and there was doubt at first about which side would succeed. When HIV first hit the public domain, the media went into overdrive, rehearsing prejudiced and stigmatising views with abandon. Yet a counter action started in the form of detailed, graphic discussion of sexual behaviour in relation to risks and prevention of HIV transmission (safer sex). This brought into the open discussions about the use of condoms for anal sex in a way that had not been seen or heard before. While exposure to these topics evoked much prejudice and criticism, it equally normalised public discussion of sexuality in general and of homosexuality in particular. A charity worker recalled these debates:

> *AIDS brought together a number of different taboos, the taboo around homosexuality, the taboo about injecting drug use, actually the taboo about dying young, and the taboos about sex and sexually transmitted infections. So, bring all that together and it is not surprising that it was such a profound, massive shock on so many levels.*

Not surprisingly, and in spite of some hopeful changes, public attitudes to homosexuality became more negative towards the end of the 1980s, after years of exposure to debates about AIDS and the perils of homosexual behaviours. The British Social Attitudes Report found that 74% of the population thought "homosexual relations to be always or mostly wrong", compared with 62% in 1983 (Jowell et al. 1988, p125). Similar findings were reported by the authors of the Wellcome Trust funded study mentioned above. The National Survey of Sexual Attitudes and Lifestyle data collected in 1990–1991 found that 70% of men thought that "gay sex was always or mostly wrong", and 64.5% "lesbian sex was always or mostly wrong" – for women the figures were 57.9% for gay sex and 58.8% for lesbian sex (Wellings et al. 1994, p271–272 and p247). Nevertheless, a hopeful sign that foretold more positive attitudes that lay ahead was easy to miss at the time. A 1988 Gallup Poll had uncovered an emergent shift of much more accepting attitudes to homosexuality amongst the under 25s (Weeks 2007, p18).

The beginning of hope and political change

The late 1990s began to bring success in the treatment of HIV, as discussed in Chapter 3. But also important political changes, with a move away from the socially conservative governments of Margaret Thatcher and John Major to more socially progressive politics with the election of the three Blair governments of 1997, 2001, and 2005. A generational change was beginning to influence social and political views. In Weeks' words, "Changes in the next decade reflected the normalization of HIV/AIDS, which became a part of the sexual landscape … Britain had conclusively moved from a society characterized by restraint to one characterized by moral pluralism and growing toleration. This was the achievement of the great transition", the generational shift that encompassed social and political change (Weeks 2007, p103 and p106). Dennis Altman saw these changes as part of a longer-reaching process: "the response to AIDS thus far has largely been a reflection of the extent to which preceding gay rights struggles had achieved a place in the political process for gay organizations; AIDS thus highlighted a process already under way" (Altman 1988, p313).

Change in public attitudes to same-sex behaviour

Compared with reports of sexual attitudes in the 1980s, increasingly more tolerant views were subsequently detected in the British population. The National Survey of Sexual Attitudes and Lifestyles collected data in 1990–1991 (Wellings et al. 1994), 1991–2001 (Johnson et al. 2001), and in 2010–2012 Mercer et al. (2013) charted the changes in attitudes to homosexuality from 1990 to 2012, showing a long arc of increased acceptance of same-sex behaviour. Amongst men, the percentage regarding male "same-sex behaviour as not wrong at all" increased from 22% to 36% and finally to 48.1%, and lesbian same-sex behaviour from 24% to 41.2%, and finally 52.4%. Amongst women, male same-sex behaviour was regarded as "not wrong at all" by 28.1%, 51.6%, and 66.3%, and lesbian behaviour as "not wrong at all" by 27.7%, 51.5%, and 66.1%. These changes were not inevitable, as one activist who was at the centre of campaigning for many years noted:

> So, what we feared in 1985, that the limited freedoms that we had started to enjoy would be taken away from us, has actually, 30 years later, developed into a quite extraordinary level of equality but, even more importantly, social attitudes completely flipped, and the response to AIDS is part of that.

What explains these changes in public attitudes, and what was the contribution of HIV to these altered perceptions of homosexual behaviour? As Weeks argues, "historians, so much better at forecasting the past than the future, did not foretell what became the defining health crisis of the time" (Weeks 2018, p.xi).

Interestingly, activists against the climate crisis have argued that "breaking the spiral of silence about climate change, much as the LGBT community did, getting as many people as possible talking about LGBT issues", is a necessary step to achieve change (Monbiot 2018; Romm 2018). Activists appearing on TV and writing in broadsheet papers, mostly articulate white men, and reports of Princess Diana's visits to hospitals and contact with PLWH ensured that AIDS was frequently in the news, and not always in a negative context. Celebrities dying as a result of HIV infection no longer provoked widespread fear, as Rock Hudson had done in 1985, but by 1991, as seen with Freddy Mercury's death in the UK in 1991, created some public sympathy towards HIV in ways that were less damning than they had been before.

It is likely that this sense of empathy and compassion spread outside hospital wards, e.g. via the AIDS quilts that memorialised the lives of the departed in moving ways. The ACT UP slogan 'Silence=Death', was in practice reversed by the public discussion of HIV and its human impact. Altman (1988) used the idea of "legitimation through disaster" to describe the effects HIV had in terms of engaging gay activists and governments and others, creating a new recognition of the gay community and movement, and the changes in public attitudes that ensued.

Legislative changes

A series of related legislative changes followed, sometimes assisted by judgements of the European Convention on Human Rights that put pressure on a hesitant British parliament. The Sexual Offences Act 2000 lowered the age of consent to 16 for both homosexual acts between men and, for the first time, for lesbian sexual acts (Northern Ireland only responded in 2009). A number of other progressive laws passed in this period that referred specifically to LGBT people, concerned the armed forces (2000), repeal of Section 28 (2003), sex discrimination (2003 and 2008) adoption (2005), assisted conception (2009), and Gender Recognition (2005). The Civil Partnership Act came into effect in 2005, recognising same-sex relations. Legislation allowing same-sex marriage, the Marriage (Same Sex Couples) Act came into force in 2014, during the socially progressive Conservative and Liberal Democrat coalition government of 2010.

Political change and more positive attitudes to LGBTQ people were a reflection of the generational changes in Britain. An HIV physician remembered:

Looking back you can see the rise of equality and diversity and LGBT rights as being enmeshed with our civil society's response to HIV, but it wasn't 'oh we have to do something good for HIV, we need to talk to more gay men', no, it was an emergence of the right people at the right time, the acceptance that you had to work together to achieve anything. So, yes, some of these things are interwoven. Certainly, AIDS made politicians talk about sex, about gay sex, about drug use, and about migration. It made people talk about things that they found uncomfortable.

The conversation that HIV charity workers had held with politicians in the 1990s did have some effect, after all, as an activist argued:

> *It is a very unfashionable thing to say today, but there were some remarkable achieve-*
> *ments of the Blair government, including the fact that I became a citizen, rather than*
> *being merely tolerated. History has been re-written to suggest that there was always*
> *consensus on gay rights, and there wasn't, the government had to spend a huge amount*
> *of political capital to equalise the age of consent and to repeal Section 28. And by the*
> *time civil partnerships came along, they did civil partnerships because they wouldn't*
> *have had the parliamentary power for same-sex marriage.*

Conclusions

While acknowledging that there has been substantial progress in terms of public acceptance of LGBTQ rights, there are some caveats worth considering. First, there is no guarantee that positive changes in public attitudes will be maintained or continue to show progress, what has been described by Weeks (2007, p4–7) as "the dangers of the Whig interpretation of sexual history". In fact, results from the 2018 British Social Attitudes Survey suggests a slight decline in tolerance towards same-sex relations (Booth 2019). The emergence of trans-exclusionary feminism is concerning. Here, a similar group of arguments against trans women are being deployed to those once reserved for gay men, e.g. as against nature/biology, aggressive and predatory (Michelson and Harrison 2020). The rise of a right-wing populist activism via social media targeting hate towards LGBTQ individuals and women, leading to an increase in physical attacks and gender-based violence is also an alarming development. While the Marriage (Same Sex Couples) Act is an achievement on one hand, some have expressed concern that the newly acquired LGBT rights may represent a new form of regulation of same-sex behaviour (Weeks 2007, p167–198; Weeks 2016, p260), or as a well-known US activist puts it: "when did our dreams get so small?, when comparing the original aims of the Gay Liberation Front with the contemporary goals of LGBTQ activism" (Duberman 2018, p66).

Clearly, we haven't reached the end of history, and the process of fighting for LGBTQ rights and winning equality continues. However, the positive impact of open discussion about HIV and its consequences, and the role of activism and developing alliances at a time when public attitudes and the political discourse were homophobic, provide lessons in how to challenge unhelpful public attitudes.

References

Alcorn K (1989) AIDS in the public sphere: how a broadcasting system in crisis dealt with an epidemic. In: Carter E and Watney S (eds) *Taking liberties: AIDS and cultural politics*. London, Serpent's Tail.

Altman D (1988) Legitimation through disaster: AIDS and the gay movement. In: Fee E and Fox DM (eds) *AIDS: The burdens of history*. Berkeley, University of California Press.

Armstrong EA and Crage SM (2006) Movements and memory: the making of the Stonewall myth. *American Sociological Review*, 71, 5, 724–751.

Booth R (2019) Public less tolerant of same-sex relations. *The Guardian*, 11 July 2019, 1–2.

Cook M (2017a) 'Archives of feeling': the AIDS crisis in Britain 1987. *History Workshop Journal*, 83, 51–78.

Cook M (2017b) AIDS, mass observation, and the fate of the permissive turn. *Journal of the History of Sexuality*, 26, 2, 239–272.

Duberman M (2018) *Has the gay movement failed?* Oakland, University of California Press.

France D (2016) *How to survive a plague: the story of how activists and scientists tamed AIDS.* London, Picador.

Hines S (2019) The feminist frontier: on trans and feminism. *Journal of Gender Studies*, 28, 2, 145–157.

Johnson A, Mercer C, Erens B, Copas A et al. (2001) Sexual behaviour in Britain: partnerships, practices, and HIV risk behaviours. *The Lancet*, 358, 1835–1842.

Johnson A, Wadsworth J, Wellings K, and Field J (1994) *Sexual attitudes and lifestyles.* Oxford, Blackwell.

Jowell R, Whitherspoon S, and Brook L (eds) (1988) *British social attitudes: the 7th report.* Aldershot, Gower.

Langhamer C (2013) *The English in love.* Oxford, Oxford University Press.

Mercer C, Tanton C, Prah P, Erens B et al. (2013) Changes in sexual attitudes and lifestyles in Britain through the life course and over time: findings from the National Surveys of Sexual Attitudes and Lifestyles (Natsal). *The Lancet*, 382, 1781–1794.

Michelson MR and Harrison BF (2020) *Transforming prejudice: identity, fear, and transgender rights.* New York, Oxford University Press.

Monbiot G (2018) While growth continues, we'll never kick our fossil fuels habit. *The Guardian*, 26 September 2018, 1–2.

Romm J (2018) The most important thing you can do to fight global warming: end the climate 'spiral of silence', https://thinkprogress.org

Watney S (1989) An introduction. In: Carter E and Watney S (eds) *Taking liberties: AIDS and cultural politics.* London, Serpent's Tail.

Weeks J (1995) *Invented moralities: sexual values in an age of uncertainty.* Cambridge, Polity Press.

Weeks J (2007) *The world we have won.* Oxon, Routledge.

Weeks J (2016) *Coming out: the emergence of LGBT identities in Britain from the 19th Century to the present* (4th edn). London, Quartet.

Weeks J (2018) *Sex, politics, and society* (4th edn) London, Routledge.

Wellings K, Field J, Johnson A, and Wadsworth J (1994) *Sexual behaviour in Britain: the national survey of sexual attitudes and lifestyles.* London, Penguin Books.

9 Prevention: What have we achieved?

Finding the way in the dark

Informal beginnings: activists, the media and public health initiatives

With the news in the early 1980s that a new, fatal and untreatable disease was spreading rapidly among gay men in the US, concerns began to be voiced in the UK, as one gay activist remembered:

> I'd worked out … the speed of the epidemic, the prevalence and the incidence meant that we were four or five, at least, years behind America and that we had this advantage. We were that much ahead in terms of prevention work.

Despite the finding in 1984 that more than a quarter of a London cohort of gay men who were being followed up for hepatitis B were already infected with HIV (Mortimer et al. 1985), it took until 1986, following the widespread attention to AIDS brought about by media reports concerning the death of Rock Hudson, for the UK government to take any action. In the words of a doctor:

> By the time the government got involved in 1986 … in a sense the horse had bolted.

What appeared to galvanise the governmental response was the fear of an explosion in heterosexual infections. It was already apparent that HIV could be spread through blood as well as through sex, and the failure to provide a safe blood supply in the UK (with heat-treated factor VIII) by the early 1980s had already led to people with haemophilia, and some people receiving blood transfusions, becoming infected with HIV.

After much debate on how the public should be alerted to HIV, the government decided to launch high-profile public information campaigns such as 'Don't Die of Ignorance' in 1987, citing risks and behaviours, but not specifically addressing the existing epidemic among gay men. These campaigns alarmed the public, as was the intent, but a male charity worker reflected on whether this approach protected gay men by not identifying them as the source of infection, or marginalised them by not addressing their needs:

> *We [assume that] the AIDS campaign 'Don't Die of Ignorance'... [in] 1987 was what changed everything. It wasn't. There had already been a fundamental change in the sex lives of most gay men before 1987 ... those who gave up sex completely, those who stopped having penetrative sex at all, [an increase in] the uptake of condom use, and its consistency ... and that was all community driven. That was before the Health Education Authority or any of the campaigns run very early on by charities.*

Just how informal gay prevention messages, not initially identifying with any formal model of health education, were able to have such an impact on gay men's sexual behaviours has been widely discussed subsequently by social scientists (King 1994). Although accurate information is clearly a pre-requisite for an informed decision to change behaviours, messages have more veracity when they come from a trusted source, as recognised by a gay activist living with HIV:

> *I got to talk to a lot of very informed people, and developed a youthful understanding of the whole notion of health education and what it takes to change and sustain behaviours, and so it's a complex but fascinating subject.*

The many gay organisations that had flourished since the gay liberation campaigns of the 1970s, including a gay press and helplines for those with issues connected to their sexuality, provided vital alerts from the US, and became foci for gay men to take on the challenges of AIDS. The importance of this community response in promoting safer sex as a fundamental aspect of gay identity early on in the epidemic, has been highlighted by community activists and academics (Watney 1989; 2013), as illustrated by a gay activist and an HIV policy maker:

> *So, activism for me was ... trying to keep the epidemic at arm's length [by] trying to sustain attachment, develop attachment, reinforce younger people's sense of belonging in this world ... in the period of Section 28 and all of that nasty, awfulness really.*

> *HIV activists in the early days were ground-breaking ... They took the initiative on prevention in their communities when the official response was slow and cautious.*

The question of mandatory testing

A major consideration within government committees was whether the spread of HIV could be limited through the screening of either the whole population or 'select groups' (Berridge 1996). Although advocated by some, the practical considerations of implementing universal testing led to much opposition. With the fear that compulsory testing could be construed as an assault on individual liberties, universal screening was never implemented. But, as an HIV policy maker recognised, the concerns of health care workers and their patients remained, with some surgeons, anaesthetists, and dentists demanding that their patients be tested before receiving treatment:

> *The British Medical Association voted in favour of the surgeons' view [that] compulsory testing of surgical patients should be permitted … There was genuine concern because it takes a while for the actual evidence to mount up that occupational transmission is rare.*

As it took up to three months for antibodies to HIV to be detectable, testing alone could never ensure the safety of health care workers. It appeared that the way forward had to be treating all patients as if they were HIV positive, i.e. taking 'universal precautions'. This soon became established practice, leading an HIV policy maker to reflect that high standards of infection control for all have become the norm, better protecting both health care workers and patients:

> *Also the education that not everyone who's infected knows they're infected so if you only take precautions for the ones you know who are infected you're not necessarily helping yourself … and of course the recently infected, the ones who are least likely to know they're infected, they might be highly viraemic too. So, you're not going to save yourself from any risk by being discriminatory about who you take precautions with.*

With fears that should a child with HIV be wounded, HIV could spread throughout a school, a paediatrician noted that universal precautions had to be adopted by all coming into contact with blood, and subsequently many unsafe practices in schools became discovered, and subsequently improved:

> *PE teachers ask, when they play rugby and they hurt themselves, we usually have a bucket and sponge and we just clean them up, do I have to stop doing that? It was basic hygiene rules which had been ignored for years. The answer was simple: well yes, you should have stopped that communal bucket and sponge long ago for health reasons, not because of HIV.*

At the same time, there was a concerted effort to educate health professionals who were not HIV specialists, and policy makers, about HIV through the recently established educational charity, the British Medical Association (BMA) Foundation for AIDS, as described by one of their administrators:

> *The BMA Foundation for AIDS was a trailblazer for an enlightened medical view on HIV, for example by informing doctors and influencing BMA policy on ethical issues such as confidentiality and consent to testing, and by encouraging GPs to test for HIV at a time when there was still reluctance among some in the HIV sector to accept testing by non-HIV specialists.*

Protecting patients from infected health care workers was also seen as important, and rather than ban all those infected from working with patients (fearing that this would be a disincentive to test or to disclose an infection), guidelines were drawn up by the Department of Health detailing practices that should be adopted, such as not performing invasive surgery, and being regularly monitored by both their treating and occupational health physician (Department of Health 1993). Despite a number of cases where infection from a health care worker to patients was considered a possibility, to date 'look-back' studies have found virtually no cases of nosocomial transmission, indicating the high level of safety afforded by universal precautions.

The complexity of prevention strategies

Beyond public education and testing: counselling and psychosocial interventions

Following the public health campaigns of 1987 there came an understanding from the government (Social Services Committee 1987) that public education through the widespread distribution of leaflets, advertisements, and media campaigns, was of limited effect, and new approaches to HIV prevention were needed.

First, a targeted approach, focusing on individual risks, was taken. In sexual health clinics, health advisers reviewed with patients ways in which they could avoid putting themselves at risk of acquiring HIV. Although practical advice was useful to many, some had difficulty in initiating and maintaining safer sex, even when they had a high knowledge of HIV transmission (Stall et al. 1990). It became clear that sexual behaviour and the meanings attached to condom use were complex, and influenced more by passion and significance than originally anticipated (Gold et al. 1991; Gold et al. 1992; Kelly et al. 1991). A gay man reflected:

> *Maybe we made errors with the prevention messages about 'you must use a condom every time' because people quickly learnt that 'oh, I didn't use a condom that time and I haven't got HIV', so they learnt it wasn't like this plus this equals this … but what [else] could you do at the time but focus on condoms because there's nothing else we had.*

As an understanding of the complexity of people's behaviours unfolded, and as more people continued to become infected, sophisticated ways of implementing prevention interventions were sought. Theories of behavioural change were applied to create new approaches in HIV prevention, and attempts made to clarify what components of behavioural interventions were important and what was redundant (Collins et al. 2014; Collins et al. 2016). As most interventions are both small and directed to specific, targeted groups, it remained difficult to prove that any one intervention is economical, efficient, and readily applicable across a wide variety of situations and client groups. However, the necessity to consider the underlying contexts implicated in risk taking, such as the prevailing economic, political, and environmental conditions, including housing, and the effects of unemployment, soon became obvious (Seeley et al. 2012; Shannon et al. 2015). A policy maker concluded that:

> *There was a lot of science of behaviour change but … [little] about the extent to which people's ability to change behaviour is constrained by society, or power structures.*

Context was particularly recognised when considering the cultural changes required of injecting drug users (Des Jarlais et al. 1986; Stimson et al. 1988). Users needed to be able to maintain safer injecting practices even when there was no available clean equipment; a particular difficulty for those injecting for the first time, or when the power dynamics of the relationship were involved, or financial transactions, could make users fearful of refusing to share unclean equipment. Recognising the complexities of safer injecting led needle exchanges not only to provide clean injecting equipment, but also to provide access to social, psychological and education services, safer sex information, items for sterilising drug equipment and condoms. So, although the possession and use of street drugs remained illegal, addressing the factors associated with HIV transmission helped to modernise drugs-related service provision, and in doing so, prevented untold harm (McKeganey and Barnard 1990), and as recognised by a gay man living with HIV:

> *Whichever Home Office or Department of Health minister authorised needle exchanges, they deserve a place in the House of Lords. The number of lives they saved.*

The criminalisation of HIV transmission

Between 1993 and 1996, discussions between the government and HIV organisations on how to reform the 1861 Offences Against the Person Act concluded that only the intentional transmission of serious infection, such as HIV, should be a criminal offence. A gay charity worker recalled:

> *THT worked hard with NAT to make sure the wording was so it avoided accidental [transmission] … but sadly the [new bill] got knocked out by an election.*

With the proposed changes never being implemented, a number of prosecutions for 'reckless' rather than 'intentional' transmission, and not in any other way illegal (such as rape, sex with a minor, coercion, or abuse), have been made under section 20 of the 1861 Act. As explained by a gay charity worker:

> *If about rape, sexual assault, there are laws that already do that. However, using the Offences Against the Person Act from [1861] is wholly inappropriate.*

An argument for maintaining the 1861 Offences Against the Person Act for transmission of HIV was that criminalisation would put the responsibility for transmission on to the person with HIV and so ensure that people don't take risks with their own or another's health. Not only did this view not reflect any shared responsibility between sexual partners, but to be found guilty of 'reckless transmission' a person needs to know their HIV positive status. A way of avoiding prosecution is, therefore, not to test. As the vast majority of HIV transmissions are from those who are undiagnosed and consequently not on antiretroviral medications, the fear of prosecution could easily increase, rather than decrease, the risk of HIV transmission, and defeat the object of using this legislation, as observed by this gay man living with HIV:

> *And there was a ridiculous state of prosecutions, which did nothing to have an impact on public health, but to turn people [away] from finding out their status, and taking medication, which would keep them alive … and make them un-infectious.*

Today, the law remains at odds with current efforts to increase the uptake of HIV testing in order that those with HIV would either adopt the rigorous use of condoms, or take antiretroviral therapy (ART) that suppresses the virus sufficiently to be untransmittable (NICE 2011). It is not clear why this Act remains. It has been suggested that attributing transmission to individuals deflects from public health failures to provide education, access to treatment, and pre-exposure prophylaxis (PrEP) (Nicholls and Rosengarten 2019).

Current situation and challenges

New infections

A gay man living with HIV observed that after more than 30 years of HIV prevention there are still 1.7 million new cases a year globally (Mahy et al. 2019), suggesting that prevention of HIV still has some way to go:

> *There hasn't been an epidemic in human history that has been controlled solely through behaviour change. They've all relied upon vaccine, or a cure, or medication.*

Despite a number of promising leads, no effective vaccine has emerged (Girard et al. 2006). But with effective medications that can prevent sexual transmissions, available to both those who are already infected and those attempting to remain uninfected, it can be asked whether the continued spread of HIV is due to ignorance, assumptions made when having unprotected sex, sharing injecting equipment, complacency, malice, fatigue or broader individual or community issues. As a charity worker recognised:

> *And we're getting new infections; we haven't got it right in terms of prevention. I think PrEP's a big issue, but I think it's just a part of it … a need to address a much more holistic picture of prevention, so to look at things like drug and alcohol use, mental health, emotional or sexual … and maybe a lot more work with the community.*

Theoretically, if all those with HIV could be identified and receive virus suppressing medication and those who are negative, engage in sex with condoms, or receive PrEP, sexual transmission would become negligible. But sufficient long-term adherence to using either condoms and/or antiretrovirals is not easy to maintain.

Facilitating effective medications

Once identified and receiving ART, a major challenge is then to enable people living with HIV (PLWH) to maintain an undetectable viral load by remaining on medication for decades. This can only be realised through continued easy access to relevant health care with ongoing psychosocial interventions to maintain adherence. Unfortunately, there is an increasing deficit between the need for, and the availability of, sexual health services that worsened in April 2020 with the removal of ring-fenced funding for public health, leading to sexual health, drug and alcohol services competing with other vital services such as social care (Gold et al. 2020).

Despite confirmation of the link between viral load and the transmissibility of HIV, resulting in the 2008 'Swiss statement' (Vernazza et al. 2008), that as long as a person has undetectable levels of virus, then they cannot transmit HIV through sexual contact, and of anecdotal evidence from San Francisco that some infected gay men were using this knowledge to abandon condoms, believing they would not infect sexual partners, prevention messages initially remained stubbornly simplistic, as described by a heterosexual man living with HIV:

> *The whole prevention thing is, wear a condom, wear a condom, wear a condom. But hang on a minute, I'm uninfectious, do I have to wear a condom, if you're with a partner who knows your status?*

It took until 2017 for a Prevention Access Campaign, 'Undetectable = Untransmittable' (U=U), that was launched the previous year by HIV activists, to be endorsed across the world by scientists and clinicians. It could be argued that a message suggesting that condoms could be abandoned was a risky one for policy makers. Once again, however, policy changes were driven by activism and U=U is now one of the key prevention messages across the globe.

When the use of ART was extended to those who had experienced a potential sexual exposure to HIV within the past 72 hours (PEP), it appeared that many who could have benefitted from PEP underestimated the risk they had taken and failed to request it (Celum et al. 2001). A gay man working with drug users, who was himself living with HIV, noted in those who did request PEP the frequent association with the use of chemsex[1]:

> *The PEP clinics we have … 33 people came for PEP that day … and 100% of them came from a chemsex background.*

Attempts to address the factors associated with the high risk sexual behaviours, leading to requests for PEP, had limited success (Llewellyn et al. 2019), neither

preventing further requests for PEP, nor the number of subsequent sexually transmitted infections. As a doctor surmised:

> *We need to focus on the people who are at risk but not infected.*

Arguments were subsequently put forward both in support of, and against, the
provision of antiretrovirals before sex, i.e. pre-exposure prophylaxis (PrEP).
Some predicted that without condoms, there would be an increase in the number of sexually transmitted infections (STIs). Interestingly, increases in both gonorrhoea and syphilis were seen (Mohammed et al. 2016; Unemo et al. 2017), but
an examination of the timings shows the rise to have begun before the introduction of PrEP. Already by 2008 the fear of infection was having less impact on
sexual behaviours. "If we're honest, we have been relying on the fear of HIV to
control sexually transmitted infections for the last 10 years," claimed Yusef Azad
(Hinsliff, 2018). It suggested that the success of ART had already led people to
be less fearful of HIV, and thus less motivated to ensure condom use in risky sex
(Crepaz et al. 2004).

NHS England notoriously promoted the idea that without the fear of HIV,
PrEP could lead to an explosion of risky sex, encourage multiple sexual partners
and become a party drug, to be used with chemsex. The Terrence Higgins Trust
(THT) accused NHS England of being "intentionally provocative and homophobic" when it said that "PrEP [is] a party drug given to people at high risk of
HIV, specifically men who have sex with men (MSM), who have condomless sex
with multiple male partners"(Iacobucci 2016). THT won the case, and MSM
instead reported the availability of PrEP decreased their anxiety and improved
their quality of life, as this comment from a doctor taking care of gay men
illustrated:

> *People who say I've not had sex for twenty years; I'm so scared of AIDS. This [PrEP]*
> *has changed my life … People [are] rediscovering their lives with this added level of*
> *protection.*

However, the admission that one is taking PrEP can be shameful. Does it indicate
a responsible attitude to sex, or suggest 'promiscuity' and 'sluttish' behaviour (Golub
et al. 2017)? Stigma makes it easier not to disclose PrEP use. A gay man living with
HIV talked of the significant impact on MSM of being able to have sex without
using a condom:

> *An old friend of mine … said he's gone on PrEP … nobody's using condoms any more,*
> *just nobody and people will say they're undetectable or they're on PrEP, but he said he*
> *can't help feeling weird, [that] having sex without a condom is unthinkable and yet it's*
> *what he's starting to do.*

It has been suggested that bringing people into the sexual health services to obtain
PrEP is an opportunity to reach men (mainly MSM) and target them with broader

health promotion messages, an opportunity frequently used with women through contraceptive and childbearing services. The benefits accruing from health promotion could offset the cost of increased numbers of health care appointments. A doctor working in an HIV clinic reflected that:

> *If it were normalised that you go for a six-month check at a, let's say, GP, rather than just going for your three-monthly sexual health checks; it's like being young, gay, sexually active doesn't mean that all your healthcare needs to be about sex … wellbeing stuff actually supports people to think about, reflect on behaviour in a positive way.*

One argument against making PrEP widely available has been its cost. Although considerable, the cost of maintaining a person infected with HIV on treatment is considerably more, and if PrEP had been more readily available in the years the NHS was suppressing treatment availability, many infections could have been prevented. A senior doctor who had worked with PLWH since the start of the epidemic highlighted how people can struggle morally with regards to PrEP:

> *You can make a case for saying that people can actually prevent being infected … so I think there is a moral question at the centre of that. As a physician, of course I think people should get the treatment but I can also see that there is a tension in people saying, well, if gay men actually were more responsible and they didn't have multiple contacts and they always used condoms then, well, we wouldn't have to spend so much money. I think it's really difficult.*

Despite the efficacy of PrEP, and its endorsement by the WHO (World Health Organisation 2015) in 2016, NHS England argued that it had the power, but not the obligation, to fund PrEP, as it is a preventative measure for those who are well, not a treatment. Frustration with this position was expressed by both a gay man living with HIV and an HIV policy maker:

> *It's a political decision not to fund [PrEP]; basically, funding people having sex; they are worried about the backlash from that. A generation ago, I think that people would have been braver.*

> *The fiasco around the commissioning of PrEP highlights the short-sightedness of separating responsibility for HIV prevention from that for HIV treatment and care.*

Repeated requests were made to the government from The Elton John AIDS Foundation, and the National AIDS Trust, amongst others, to ensure that PrEP is available to all who need it. Only in the spring of 2020 did they achieve an assurance that PrEP would be provided through local authorities across England to anyone who is at high risk of contracting HIV, a triumph articulated by Ian Green, Chief Executive of the Terrence Higgins Trust, who said "This is an historic day in the context of the HIV epidemic. It comes after years of fighting, campaigning and lobbying" (O'Shea 2020). In the process of achieving access to PrEP, a new wave of activism was sparked, a view echoed by an HIV policy maker and a gay man living with HIV:

> *[The activists] legacy lives on in the resurgence of grassroots campaigning for access to PrEP, the role of community-based organisations in providing information and peer support to people living with HIV and the recognition by the NHS of the importance of patient and public involvement.*

> *There was such opposition to the idea of PrEP ... that created a new activism ... a whole bunch of younger gay men started coming out of the woodwork and, lo and behold, there's new energy in the field of sexual health, bringing together PLWH and medics.*

Neglected populations: ethnic and minority groups, women, migrants and injecting drug users

With the advent of ART and PrEP, the fight against HIV should be drawing to a close. In reality, education and medication are not available to all, and enabling access is fraught with issues, moral, practical, and economic, as highlighted by a doctor in 2019:

> *If the assumption from governments and the general public is that HIV is fixed, well ... we still have a group of vulnerable people, be they migrants, people without much money, gay men, transgendered people, who are vulnerable for numerous reasons.*

Historically, the main UK government health campaigns failed to target certain communities of high risk, such as African groups (Scott-Clark and Levy 2005), as a charity worker observed:

> *The prevention needs [are] woefully inadequate for African communities, for sexual health for gay men. Prevention activities [are] grossly underfunded and poorly coordinated.*

Targeted campaigns have reported some success, such as a decline in new infections in Black African adults being seen since 2015. However, we still need to address the factors that result in 60% of heterosexual men and 52% of Black African adults being diagnosed late (Public Health England 2019), a situation that both increases the damage HIV has on health, and the likelihood that the infection has spread to others (Lodi et al. 2011).

At the time of writing this book, generic, off-patent PrEP was available on-line and could be purchased from a progressive sexual health clinic in London. But its use was mainly being taken up in affluent white communities, particularly by

MSM, and less so by Black MSM. A gay man living with HIV recognised that the major challenge now, is how to spread its use to all at risk of being infected:

> *The people who are currently getting PrEP are the well informed, 30 and 40 year olds; well educated, largely white, largely employed gay men, so now … it's the disadvantaged people who need to be getting it.*

One group who could benefit from PrEP is pregnant women in discordant couples (where the man has HIV) (Zorrilla et al. 2018), as most of the infants now born with HIV are to women with positive partners, resulting from condomless sex during pregnancy, a time when contraception is no longer required. Another frequently overlooked group is migrants. In the UK most migrants, including many women, come from sub-Saharan or West Africa. It appears that most infection occurs post migration (Alvarez-del Arco et al. 2017; Pantazis et al. 2019), suggesting that there continue to be barriers to testing and subsequent care, in the UK (del Amo 2019).

Conclusions

For more than 30 years substantial efforts have been made to prevent ongoing transmission of HIV. Without doubt, many infections have been prevented, but although praised (as by this charity worker) could more have been done, and what is still required?

> *Oh, it's utterly transformed … We have continued to maintain the safety of the blood supply, big success. We were a bit slower on really preventing mother to child transmission but now a big, massive success. However, the big challenges are continued transmission, particularly amongst gay men, but also heterosexual transmission.*

The initial universal prevention campaign in the 1980s certainly brought knowledge of HIV to the majority of the population, but it was criticised for not targeting the specific risk group of gay men, who were most affected. The reduction in unsafe sex in gay men in the 1980s, a major behaviour change, predated the government's first response and can be attributed to the critical efforts of gay activists and voluntary groups.

The government initially embraced the knowledge and involvement of gay activists and community groups, in devising prevention activities, but as it professionalised health education, gay groups were mainly excluded from prevention campaigns. As King states (King 1994), "It is now clear that in practice the de-gaying of the epidemic worked to gay men's disadvantage, in that it marginalised their concerns and obstructed the provision of ongoing safer sex campaigns". A gay professional commented on the issue:

> *Well, the tombstones and the icebergs were actually not very helpful, because they prompted fear rather than knowledge. A lot of the advertising that has subsequently been*

done by people like THT is specifically targeted at groups in the population who are at greatest risk, doing it in their language and in ways that they're going to think 'Oh yes, there's a point there', so I think we need to continue to take advice from the voluntary sector about how best to get these sorts of messages across.

With the current emphasis on 'treatment as prevention', rapid diagnoses and early identification of HIV status are required. Remaining undiagnosed is not only unhelpful for an individual's health, but it provides increased opportunities for people to unwittingly infect others, thus putting the spotlight on the socioeconomic reality of disadvantaged communities. Structural interventions to reduce stigma and poverty and increase the accessibility of healthcare are required (Bereczky 2019); a position endorsed by a doctor:

We need to look at better ways to make sure that everyone who is either non infected and at risk of HIV infection or who is HIV positive, has equality of access to services that can help reduce their risk, help support behaviour change … At the moment I feel that's becoming very inequitable.

Additionally, we need to identify factors that increase sexual risk taking, and implement interventions to address them. Studies emphasise the need for multi-agency working that promotes collaboration and integration between HIV, mental health, alcohol, and substance abuse services (Nöstlinger et al. 2020).

With a new stream of young adults starting their sex lives each year it would seem obvious that HIV prevention messages need to be maintained and updated throughout the epidemic, including in schools. This seems to have been overlooked or neglected. Recognising that years of inaction in education and prevention campaigns have failed to protect new generations of adults, a gay activist living with HIV and a charity worker commented:

Education is a challenge that needs to be repeated and repeated, and is on-going as every generation becomes more and more sexually [active].

I think the political failures, things we've got wrong, sex education in schools, campaigning for it for 30 years and it's still not there.

The 1980s prevention campaign targeted every household with leaflets. Now, with the internet and social media, maybe there are more efficient ways to promote testing (Hatzold et al. 2019). Ideas of how to engage young people using technology, and techniques developed by advertisers, such as linking prevention tips to Apps such as Grindr, could provide the necessary information just when people need it (Hightow-Weidman 2019). The experience of a gay man working with drug users indicated some of the difficulties:

HIV prevention is getting so much more complicated; understanding undetectable viral loads … PrEP … PEP, as well as condoms … let alone managing Grindr; how to write their profiles … your sexual needs and how to communicate them.

With recent cuts to the health prevention budgets, a charity worker and a doctor reflected that it is unlikely that if all those at risk took up the required services, there would be sufficient resources:

> *So when people stopped dying by and large, the number of people with AIDS grew, and that created twin challenges of needing to do more on prevention because you had a growing number of people living with HIV and growing pressure on services that had become crucially, very underfunded because there was a decline in public visibility and engagement with AIDS issues and the big drop in funding for social care and prevention.*

> *Politicians are in for the short haul … and the fact that people who aren't going to be there in 5 years' time who are taking political decisions means that of course the cost–benefit analysis is overwhelming, but these calculations are not seen as important as they should be.*

To make an impact on the HIV epidemic, PrEP implementation needs to be large-scale, targeted, and rapid. Attempts are being made to increase knowledge and interest in PrEP to all those at risk, not solely white MSM (National AIDS Trust 2018) and to reduce the stigma associated with its use (Golub 2018). Innovative approaches are needed to support the less organised lifestyle of some drug users, and to assess and treat problematic sexualised drug use among PrEP users (Sewell et al. 2018). As a gay activist remarked:

> *[Prevention] is not won at all. There's a myth that it's won. Yes, we're winning … but you have to have everything set up just right, and it's not just PrEP. You have to do something that means people come in and test regularly … and it's got to be fast. Whether it's PrEP or whether it's HIV treatment, they've got to walk out of the clinic door, with the pills in their pocket on the first appointment.*

There are concerns about the unintended consequences of U=U and PrEP, as raised by a senior doctor, in particular, whether the abandonment of condoms would lead to an increase in STIs or set the scene for a future viral epidemic:

> *Is [HIV] just preventable by treatment, or PrEP, or is it preventable by behaviour? Or, in the absence of a vaccine, is PrEP a solution to the demand for a lifestyle immune from the HIV and if, as a public health view is that then going to lead to the next behaviourally determined epidemic in 2030, who knows?*

The radical approach of harm minimisation, adopted in the 1980s towards injecting drug users proved wise and as services for IDUs changed, many users survived. But the recent increase in HIV infection seen in drug users has been linked with cuts to public health budgets (National AIDS Trust 2018) where recent innovations such as Drug Consumption Rooms, (that provide a safe, clean environment for injecting), have been closed. Changes in the management of IDU appear to have been driven by political decisions, and the success of adopting a harm minimisation approach seems to have been forgotten, as an HIV service developer clearly recognised:

> *Drug services had to reconfigure and had to say this group aren't dying, where do we go now, and what does this mean for the next generation of drug users? … in the last few years things got difficult, because of austerity and cutbacks and people not remembering that history … the recovery agenda has taken over, recovery being the code word for abstinence, and it started when the current government started revamping the policy. It took a lot of hard work to try and get them to acknowledge the fact that some people weren't going to become abstinent … There was a paradigm shift towards recovery, and you can't argue that we don't want recovery, so everyone was caught up a little in this bind, we were characterised as being of the old-fashioned approach of just drugging people up with methadone and not recognising people's potential. It is hard not to be political, because you see every government screwing up with drug users.*

It appears that we have the tools to end the epidemic but as recognised by a gay charity worker and a gay nurse, the political, economic, and health care systems are not yet supporting necessary access, such as testing, immediate treatment, and ongoing monitoring to bring HIV prevention to many communities:

> *There's a real opportunity to knock [HIV] on the head … more testing to flush out those people who have got HIV and don't know it who are obviously the drivers of the epidemic and PrEP to protect those people who find it difficult to use condoms all the time and are in high risk situations.*

> *Like the trans community who are not accessing services, because of some poor treatment by health services … they get an appalling deal.*

As, to date, no successful vaccine has been developed, HIV prevention remains complicated. It is not a question of condoms or treatment, as both can be very effective when used correctly and are available and affordable. Behaviours directly linked to virus transmission can be modified, e.g. being abstinent, selecting HIV uninfected sexual partners, being monogamous with an HIV uninfected partner, engaging in safer sex and avoiding sharing equipment for injecting drugs. Alternatively, or additionally, advantage can be taken of PrEP, or, if positive, reducing one's own infectivity through maintaining an undetectable viral load. It appears that effective prevention needs to look beyond the narrow focus on HIV risk and integrate PrEP into a combination prevention approach (De Boni et al. 2018; Pinto et al. 2018), addressing issues such as drug use, depression and sexual risk (Nöstlinger et al. 2020).

On an optimistic note, with testing and treating those already infected, and the use of either PrEP or condoms together with initiatives and sufficient resources to maintain adherence, HIV could be eliminated, but as a gay activist living with HIV cautioned:

> *If you want to increase an epidemic, you cut funding for prevention.*

Note

1 Chemsex usually means the use of mephedrone, γ-hydroxybutyrate [GHB], γ-butyrolactone [GBL], and/or methamphetamine to heighten sexual pleasure and reduce challenging feelings.

References

Alvarez-del Arco, D, Fakoya, I, Thomadakis, C, Pantazis, N, Touloumi, G, Gennotte, A-F,… Göpel, S (2017) High levels of postmigration HIV acquisition within nine European countries. *AIDS*, 31(14), 1979–1988.

Bereczky, T (2019) U = U is a blessing: but only for patients with access to HIV treatment: an essay by Tamás Bereczky. *BMJ*, 366, l5554.

Berridge, V (1996) *AIDS in the UK: The Making of a Policy, 1981–1994*. Oxford, Oxford University Press.

Celum, CL, Buchbinder, SP, Donnell, D, Douglas Jr, JM, Mayer, K, Koblin, B,… Flores, J (2001) Early human immunodeficiency virus (HIV) infection in the HIV Network for prevention trials vaccine preparedness cohort: risk behaviors, symptoms, and early plasma and genital tract virus load. *The Journal of Infectious Diseases*, 183(1), 23–35.

Collins, LM, Trail, JB, Kugler, KC, Baker, TB, Piper, ME, and Mermelstein, RJ (2014) Evaluating individual intervention components: making decisions based on the results of a factorial screening experiment. *Translational Behavioral Medicine*, 4(3), 238–251.

Collins, LM, Kugler, KC, and Gwadz, MV (2016) Optimization of multicomponent behavioral and biobehavioral interventions for the prevention and treatment of HIV/AIDS. *AIDS and Behavior*, 20(1), 197–214.

Crepaz, N, Hart, TA, and Marks, G (2004) Highly active antiretroviral therapy and sexual risk behavior: a meta-analytic review. *JAMA*, 292(2), 224–236.

De Boni, RB, Machado, IK, De Vasconcellos, MT, Hoagland, B, Kallas, EG, Madruga, JV,… Goulart, SP (2018) Syndemics among individuals enrolled in the PrEP Brasil Study. *Drug and Alcohol Dependence*, 185, 168–172.

del Amo, J (2019) *HIV infection in migrant populations in Europe; changes and challenges. Paper presented at the AIDS Imact: 14th International Conference*, London.

Department of Health (1993) *AIDS and HIV infected health care workers: guidance on the management of infected health care workers (interim)*. London, Department of Health.

Des Jarlais, DC, Friedman, SR, and Strug, D (1986) AIDS and needle sharing within the IV-drug use subculture. In Feldman, Douglas A., and Thomas M. Johnson (eds) *The social dimensions of AIDS: Method and theory* (pp. 111–125). New York, Praeger.

Girard, MP, Osmanov, SK, and Kieny, MP (2006) A review of vaccine research and development: the human immunodeficiency virus (HIV). *Vaccine*, 24(19), 4062–4081.

Gold, RS, Skinner, MJ, Grant, PJ, and Plummer, DC (1991) Situational factors and thought processes associated with unprotected intercourse in gay men. *Psychology and Health*, 5(4), 259–278.

Gold, RS, Karmiloff-Smith, A, Skinner, MJ, and Morton, J (1992) Situational factors and thought processes associated with unprotected intercourse in heterosexual students. *AIDS Care*, 4(3), 305–323.

Gold, D, Green, I, and Carlin, E (2020) Sexual health services must be protected to prevent a crisis. *The Observer*.

Golub, SA (2018) PrEP stigma: implicit and explicit drivers of disparity. *Current HIV/AIDS Reports*, 15(2), 190–197.

Golub, SA, Gamarel, KE, and Surace, A (2017) Demographic differences in PrEP-related stereotypes: implications for implementation. *AIDS and Behavior*, 21(5), 1229–1235.

Hatzold, K, Gudukeya, S, Mutseta, MN, Chilongosi, R, Nalubamba, M, Nkhoma, C,… Mabhunu, V (2019) HIV self-testing: breaking the barriers to uptake of testing among men and adolescents in sub-Saharan Africa, experiences from STAR demonstration projects in Malawi, Zambia and Zimbabwe. *Journal of the International AIDS Society*, 22, e25244.

Hightow-Weidman, L (2019) *Innovations in mobile technology for maximising youth engagement and behaviour change in HIV treatment and prevention interventions*. Paper presented at the *AIDSImpact 14th International Conference*, London.

Hinsliff, G (2018) Dangerous liaisons: why syphilis and gonorrhoea have returned to haunt Britain, *Guardian* 24 July 2018, https://www.theguardian.com/society/2018/jul/23/dangerous-liaisons-why-syphilis-and-gonorrhea-have-returned-to-haunt-britain

Iacobucci, G (2016, August 8) HIV Charity criticises NHS England over 'homophobic' PrEP statement, *British Medical Journal*, 354, i4347.

Kelly, J, Kalichman, SC, Kauth, MR, Kilgore, HG, Hood, HV, Campos, PE, … St Lawrence, JS (1991) Situational factors associated with AIDS risk behavior lapses and coping strategies used by gay men who successfully avoid lapses. *American Journal of Public Health*, 81(10), 1335–1338.

King, E (1994) *Safety in numbers: Safer sex and gay men*, New York, Routledge.

Llewellyn, CD, Abraham, C, Pollard, A, Jones, CI, Bremner, S, Miners, A, and Smith, H (2019) A randomised controlled trial of a telephone administered brief HIV risk reduction intervention amongst men who have sex with men prescribed post-exposure prophylaxis for HIV after sexual exposure in the UK: Project PEPSE. *PLoS One*, 14(5), e0216855.

Lodi, S, Phillips, A, Touloumi, G, Geskus, R, Meyer, L, Thiébaut, R, Babiker, A et al. … (2011) Time from human immunodeficiency virus seroconversion to reaching CD4+ cell count thresholds<200,< 350, and < 500 cells/mm3: assessment of need following changes in treatment guidelines. *Clinical Infectious Diseases*, 53(8), 817–825.

Mahy, M, Marsh, K, Sabin, K, Wanyeki, I, Daher, J, and Ghys, PD (2019) *HIV estimates through 2018: data for decision-making*. In: *AIDS 2019*, Supp 3: S203–S211.

McKeganey, N, and Barnard, M (1990) Drug injectors' risks for HIV. In *AIDS: Individual, Cultural And Policy Dimensions* (pp. 151–162), Abingdon, Routledge Falmer.

Mohammed, H, Mitchell, H, Sile, B, Duffell, S, Nardone, A, and Hughes, G (2016) Increase in sexually transmitted infections among men who have sex with men, England, 2014. *Emerging Infectious Diseases*, 22(1), 88.

Mortimer, P, Jesson, W, Vandervelde, E, and Pereira, M (1985) Prevalence of antibody to human T lymphotropic virus type III by risk group and area, United Kingdom 1978–84. *British Medical Journal (Clinical Research Ed.)*, 290(6476), 1176–1178.

National AIDS Trust (2018) *Policy Briefing: HIV Outbreak in Glasgow – more needs to be done*. London, National AIDS Trust.

NICE (2011) *NICE public health guidance 34 Increasing the uptake of HIV testing to reduce undiagnosed infection and prevent transmission among men who have sex with men*. London, National Institute for Health and Clinical Excellence.

Nicholls, EJ, and Rosengarten, M (2019) Witness seminar: the criminalisation of HIV transmission in the UK. https://research.gold.ac.uk/26769/1/criminalisation_WS_Published.pdf

Nöstlinger, C, Reyniers, T, Smekens, T, Apers, H, Laga, M, Wouters, K, and Vuylsteke, B (2020) Drug use, depression and sexual risk behaviour: a syndemic among early pre-exposure prophylaxis (PrEP) adopters in Belgium? *AIDS Care*, 32 1–8.

O'Shea, D [Medscape] (2020, 17 March) HIV PrEP to be made available across England. https://www.medscape.com/viewarticle/926891

Pantazis, N, Thomadakis, C, del Amo, J, Alvarez-del Arco, D, Burns, FM, Fakoya, I, and Touloumi, G (2019) Determining the likely place of HIV acquisition for migrants in Europe combining subject-specific information and biomarkers data. *Statistical Methods in Medical Research*, 28(7), 1979–1997.

Pinto, R M, Berringer, K R, Melendez, R, and Mmeje, O (2018) Improving PrEP implementation through multilevel interventions: a synthesis of the literature. *AIDS and Behavior*, 22(11), 3681–3691.

Public Health England (2019) *Trends in new HIV diagnoses and in people receiving HIV-related care in the United Kingdom: data to the end of December 2018*. London, Public Health England.

Scott-Clark, C, and Levy, A (2005) Where it's really hurting. *The Guardian Weekend*.

Seeley, J, Watts, CH, Kippax, S, Russell, S, Heise, L, and Whiteside, A (2012) Addressing the structural drivers of HIV: a luxury or necessity for programmes? *Journal of the International AIDS Society*, 15, 17397.

Sewell, J, Cambiano, V, Miltz, A, Speakman, A, Lampe, FC, Phillips, A, … Nwokolo, N (2018) Changes in recreational drug use, drug use associated with chemsex, and HIV-related behaviours, among HIV-negative men who have sex with men in London and Brighton, 2013–2016. *Sexually Transmitted Infections*, 94(7), 494–501.

Shannon, K, Strathdee, SA, Goldenberg, SM, Duff, P, Mwangi, P, Rusakova, M, … Pickles, MR (2015) Global epidemiology of HIV among female sex workers: influence of structural determinants. *The Lancet*, 385(9962), 55–71.

Social Services Committee (1987) *Problems Associated with AIDS*. London, HMSO.

Stall, R, Ekstrand, M, Pollack, L, McKusick, L, and Coates, TJ (1990) Relapse from safer sex: the next challenge for AIDS prevention efforts. *Journal of Acquired Immune Deficiency Syndromes*, 3(12), 1181–1187.

Stimson, GV, Alldritt, L, Dolan, K, and Donoghoe, M (1988) Syringe exchange schemes for drug users in England and Scotland. *British Medical Journal (Clinical Research Ed.)*, 296(6638), 1717–1719.

Unemo, M, Bradshaw, CS, Hocking, JS, de Vries, HJ, Francis, SC, Mabey, D, … Hoornenborg, E (2017) Sexually transmitted infections: challenges ahead. *The Lancet Infectious Diseases*, 17(8), e235–e279.

Vernazza, P, Hirschel, B, Bernasconi, E, and Flepp, M (2008) HIV-positive individuals without additional sexually transmitted diseases (STD) and on effective anti-retroviral therapy are sexually non-infectious. *Bulletin des médecins suisses*, 89, 165–169.

Watney, S (1989) A common tragedy: the politics of AIDS. *Gay Times*, 130, 42–45.

Watney, S (2013) Safer sex as community practice. In *AIDS: Individual, cultural and policy dimensions* (pp. 27–42). Abingdon, Routledge.

World Health Organisation (2015) *Policy brief: pre-exposure prophylaxis (PrEP): WHO expands recommendation on oral pre-exposure prophylaxis of HIV infection (PrEP)*. Geneva, WHO.

Zorrilla, CD, Báez, FR, Colón, KG, Ibarra, J, García, I, and Mosquera, AM (2018) HIV seroconversion during pregnancy and the need for pre-exposure prophylaxis (PrEP). *HIV/AIDS (Auckland, NZ)*, 10, 57.

10 Conclusions and future challenges

What did our participants tell us?

Our research focused on the way care, support, and efforts to prevent the spread of HIV developed and evolved over the years. We traced the UK HIV epidemic from the early realisation that a serious new illness had arrived on the scene, through to the awareness of a new viral cause, and the growing sense of importance of the emerging epidemic. We covered in detail the first-hand, frequently moving experiences of HIV infection, illnesses, and how the NHS, activists, and communities organised to cope as best they could under difficult circumstances, and not without hostility from the wider community. The creative and political solutions that subsequently arose, the prioritising of people's humanity in the care approaches developed, and the solidarity and sense of collaborative effort that developed between people living with HIV (PLWH) and their formal and informal carers, were features of the narratives we collected. We followed the epidemic right through to the current era of biomedically successful treatments and the mainstreaming of services for PLWH, where HIV has come to be treated as a more ordinary, long-term condition by many, albeit with some recognition that this may never be so.

We argue that the complex threads of HIV care came together in the UK in such a way that one of the first truly multidisciplinary and person-centred health care services was established by the NHS. By all accounts, HIV care was not just a *rhetoric* about the value of focusing on individual needs. Instead, HIV care became an actual incubator for a radical re-imagining of health care that elevated patient experience in a way that was without precedent for the state health service. A change that would anticipate – and gradually usher in a new NHS discourse about personalisation – including the idea that patients could be more involved in – as well as allowed increasing control of – their care (de Iongh et al. 2019). Nevertheless, we also contend that subsequently, with the arrival of effective biomedical treatments, and without the high level of challenge presented by a newly stigmatised, sexualised and inevitably deadly condition, there was a gradual drift back towards the biomedical model of care. Along with the pressures of cost cutting, HIV care subsequently integrated back into the NHS mainstream, and a re-medicalisation of care ensued.

The first five chapters explore the experience of HIV from the early 1980s to date. Chapter 1 highlighted how 1980s Britain – influenced by gay liberation and feminism – was increasingly a socially and sexually progressive society, yet with a core conservative ruling class. This new landscape not only made the UK vulnerable to the initial spread of the virus, but also adept at mobilising a highly effective resistance and response to initial HIV complacency. Activists piled on pressure and inspired a sluggish government, eventually compelling influential members to act to better protect the communities affected. Here, we saw how some remarkable people, whether from the coalface of the epidemic or the political elite, began to collaborate and deal humanely (rather than reactively) with the extraordinary existential threat posed by the virus. To a degree, these people moved in a counter direction to the tide of stigma and negative attitudes in sections of the media and community, who frankly lacked compassion. Thus, activists, young medical trainees, nurses, clinical psychologists, and experienced doctors were thrown together to respond as best they could to this unprecedented challenge. Professionals – who brought fresh thinking to the NHS – found themselves in the HIV sector for varying reasons, such as being part of affected communities, intellectual curiosity or just having a keen sense of social justice. This historic synergy resulted in a truly person-centred care, probably at least partly because effective treatments were lacking at the time.

Chapter 2 outlined how the affected communities and activists, the NHS, political elites, and charities began to respond to HIV early on in the epidemic. They built alliances and coordinated efforts at public awareness campaigning, gay community safer sex campaigning, harm minimisation approaches in drug-using populations, as well as funded care for PLWH (e.g. complementary therapies to ease suffering). Additionally, it became clear that celebrities were not immune to HIV, which raised the public profile of the virus, and garnered more measured public sympathy for PLWH. HIV testing also became widely available, obviously a critical development in prevention and care, although a positive HIV result was a disturbing forewarning of impending death. By now, the full horror of HIV was unfolding, not only in terms of the level of stigmatisation of people with AIDS that needed to be challenged, but also with the increasing deaths that previously fit, (frequently) young men and their carers (often of similar ages to PLWH) endured. While some deaths were peaceful, the memories of terrible deaths haunted those we interviewed. The trauma for PLWH, their loved ones and carers was considerable, and still tangible in many of our interviews. The NHS and charities attempted to cope as best they could. HIV-specific hospices were set up to cater not just for end of life care, but also to provide respite with the recurrent illnesses associated with AIDS, and so promote better quality of life for both PLWH and their carers.

As outlined in Chapter 3, the years from 1988 to 1995 involved painfully slow progress in treatment development, although a promising emerging global response to AIDS consolidated. There were regular International AIDS Conferences, and the World Health Organisation's Global Programme on AIDS was developed. At the same time, the epidemic in the UK broadened out from gay men to include Black African men and women. Better treatments for opportunistic infections emerged, as did antiretrovirals (but with invariably disappointing longer-term results) as the virus quickly mutated and became resistant to the medications. Side effects could be severe, and it was not a straightforward decision for PLWH to try the new medications. ACT UP emerged to push for early access to better treatments; celebrities became more involved in publicly fighting for AIDS; we learned that not all health workers were above stigmatising attitudes; and compensation to people with haemophilia who had contracted HIV through contaminated supplies of factor VIII was finally made available in the UK. And while the epidemic continued to spread (including increasingly among white heterosexuals, and newborns), the needs of all affected by HIV were attended to as awareness of their issues improved. The person-centredness of the services – and continuity of care – both moved and surprised some groups (e.g. substance users who were less used to being well treated by health professionals). HIV care was clearly set apart from mainstream health in this era, and not without resentment from other areas of the medical establishment.

Chapter 4 traced the increasing success of combination antiretroviral therapies, which although – heartbreakingly – too late for many PLWH, and initially more toxic than current-day regimens, gradually led to significant improvements in health. As morbidity and mortality dramatically fell over time, the person-centred approach established in HIV care at a time of limited treatment successes, came under strain. Care became increasingly focused on managing medication and its technical and practical aspects. While person-centredness survived to a degree, for many it seemed as if HIV care was drifting back to a more traditional medical model. Not just because of pharmacological treatment, but also as the wider political winds changed. While for the media and in much public discourse, HIV ceased to be a crisis, difficulties with everyday living continued for PLWH, as many continued to battle grief, as well as physical and mental health problems. After an extended period of dedicated service, charity workers and professionals who had been at the coalface of the epidemic, began to down tools and take on other professional roles or new challenges.

In Chapter 5, we outlined how the epidemic changed from 2010 to the current day, where HIV came to be seen as more akin to living with a long-term health condition. At the same time, the financial crash of 2008 ushered in an ideological era of brutal cuts to health care and other social services, hastening the decline in person-centred HIV care. But this was also the time when simplified 'once a day' medical regimens emerged, promoting increased adherence, and a more advanced scientific understanding of HIV – especially in terms of treatment-related prevention – began to usher in new hopes for halting the HIV epidemic. While quality of life dramatically improved for many PLWH, others continued to struggle with co-morbidities and their mental health, while also dealing with persistent stigma, and a new sense of abandonment as their NHS HIV specialist services wound down. Despite the upheavals of this period, it became clear that people newly diagnosed with HIV were to have largely better experiences than the initial cohort infected, despite increasingly fragmented care, and a difficult funding environment for the NHS and charities. As the decade drew to a close, a new activism around pre-exposure prophylaxis (PrEP) helped to create hope that the epidemic might one day end.

The next four chapters discussed key issues that emerged in our research. Chapter 6 explored the development of HIV care as a unique example of the emergence of a person-centred model of care. While it was not the first time that this model of care had been advocated, its implementation is recognised by our participants as one of the defining – perhaps even revolutionary – features of a particularly tragic episode in health care in the UK. Here, doctors and nurses aspired to a kind of care which included the views of PLWH as fundamental to decision making, and HIV became a living example of how personalised care could be achieved in practice. While HIV care anticipated current-day rhetoric (if not practices) of person-centred care, it remains to be seen if there is the political will to reinvent the NHS in this direction.

Chapter 7 explored the close – and continuing – connection between death and HIV from the start of the epidemic, through to successful treatments and beyond. The initial impact of (mostly) young men and drug users dying from HIV was powerful in shaping UK responses to the epidemic. As the epidemic changed, it was influenced by wider neoliberal discourses, particularly as discourses about how citizens (rather than the state) should take responsibility – and action – to improve their health proliferated. Here, 'successful ageing' became an allied discourse. Our chapter highlighted that HIV deaths were initially experienced as traumatic and devastating, but also potentially energising, leading to highly creative responses. After the introduction of effective therapies, dying changed shape, it had not disappeared, with those presenting late and/or with co-morbidities continuing to die. Participants drew attention to the ways in which people died, with a new – potentially deadly – chemsex epidemic emerging among gay men, and via the ageing of informal and formal carers who were now themselves retiring or dying.

Chapter 8 explored the changing attitudes to sex and sexuality in connection to the HIV epidemic. We argued that HIV pushed sexual minorities and varying sexual practices into the spotlight, and so worked to place stories into the mainstream in a way that humanised minorities. While we acknowledge substantial progress in terms of public acceptance of lesbian, gay, bisexual, trans and queer identifying (LGBTQ) people and their rights, there are some caveats worth noting. First, there is no guarantee that positive changes in public attitudes will be maintained or continue to show progress. We presented some evidence of a decline in tolerance towards same-sex relations in the UK, as well as the potential new regulation of same-sex behaviours, such as via the new activism for equal marriage rights.

Chapter 9 focused on the many facets of HIV prevention. It was community activists who, in a sense, invented safer sex early on in the epidemic, resisting calls for draconian, anti-sex approaches to limit the spread of HIV. While the government led on some public health education, community groups had already developed safer sex and injecting drug use information and campaigns that best resonated with their communities. Once the complexities of risk behaviours were better understood, it was clear that multi-layered approaches were needed, including adapting theories of behavioural change to interventions and provision of needle exchanges and targeting counselling and psychological services to support vulnerable people. Some interventions such as the criminalisation of HIV transmission were less useful. Biomedical interventions, including treatment as prevention and PrEP, which is now available through the NHS, have contributed to a range of options to reduce risk, and decreased transmission of HIV among gay men. As always, there are social and moral issues connected with biomedical options, such as the lack of access to PrEP among those most vulnerable to HIV (including Black and ethnic minority men) (Nagington and Sandset 2020), and the increased complexities of negotiating risk reduction under conditions of ongoing stigma, homophobia and the growing range of preventative options available (e.g. condoms, treatment as prevention, PrEP).

What have we learnt? Drawing up the lessons from the UK epidemic

Scanning across our findings on the lived experience of the UK HIV epidemic, we have drawn together what we believe to be some of the key lessons.

First, it is clear that the role of community activists at all stages, in initiating, developing, and adapting approaches to the epidemic was – and remains – crucial. Even as HIV became re-medicalised in more recent times, a new activism emerged that forced the government after a five-year battle, to make PrEP available through the NHS.

Second, the role of charities was crucial in the fight for a just and humane response to HIV. Charities like the Terrence Higgins Trust and the National AIDS Trust played crucial roles in making PrEP freely available on the NHS. The National AIDS Trust, for example, campaigned to limit the detrimental impact of prosecutions for reckless transmission of HIV, e.g. by working with authorities, and intervening on a case-by-case basis in the justice system. The London Lighthouse and the Mildmay Mission hospice are other examples of charities that played an enormous part in providing education, care, and support to PLWH and their friends and families.

Third, with roots in the liberation movements of the 1960s, especially gay liberation, the formation of alliances between communities most affected by HIV, PLWH, the healthcare services and charity workers, the Department of Health and other parts of government was critical in battling stigma, optimising the treatment of PLWH, and enabling prevention efforts. Rose (2007) has described the alliance developed between AIDS activists and the biomedical community as 'exemplary' in terms of its achievements.

Fourth, HIV became a model of how to address complex issues, from how to involve patients and the public in research, and ways in which specific health conditions could be re-imagined, such as via activism to push forward treatments for dementia, to promote the rights of people with disabilities and mental health issues, through to approaches to decrease global warming. HIV highlighted the critical importance of telling and hearing human stories as a vital first step to attracting people's interest in a marginalised issue and gaining political traction for a cause. If ACT UP was right that SILENCE = DEATH, then it could be said that TALKING = LIFE. HIV showed that giving voice to excluded individuals, their ideas and needs, regardless of how they are perceived or stigmatised within society, can help a marginalised narrative to prevail, thus prioritising our common humanity.

Challenges ahead

Despite the positive social changes made through HIV prevention and care initiatives, here we follow up just a few of the challenges identified by our participants that remain to be met. While we interviewed women living with HIV and women at the forefront of managing the epidemic, women are still overly invisible in our stories about experiences of HIV. We tried to include more voices of women in our study, and 3 in 10 participants were women, however, most women we interviewed were professionals. Women make up a third of all those diagnosed, yet we know little about what living with HIV is like for women, what their specific needs are, nor how to best support them from infection (Bell et al. 2018). The neglect of women's health needs is not unique to HIV. Criado-Perez (2019) argues that the world is generally built around research focusing on men, and the results can be disastrous for women. For example, when female symptoms for a heart attack (e.g. fatigue, sweating rather than crushing chest pain) look so different to predominantly documented male patterns, they can be overlooked by health professionals. There is a great deal of work to do to bring women's data and voices into research and policy.

Encouragingly, people over 50 in the UK who have HIV now have a longer life expectancy than ever before. People are ageing with HIV, as well as increasingly acquiring HIV in later life. Some European countries estimate that over 70% of PLWH will be aged 50 or over by 2030 (Sherr et al. 2016). However, a survey of PLWH by the Terrence Higgins Trust (2017) found that nearly 6 in 10 participants over 50 lived below (or just on) the poverty line, while around 8 in 10 worried about how they would care for – and finance themselves – in the future. There is relatively little time to adapt to the health and social needs of ageing PLWH. There are many challenges that older PLWH face, including HIV stigma, ageism, poorer health related to HIV and other health conditions, and difficulties gaining appropriate long-term social support (Rosenfeld et al. 2019). For older LGBTQ people, inequalities are especially apparent in formal social care settings, where homophobia endangers identities, social relations, and lives (Kneale et al. 2019).

An increase in drug-user deaths in Scotland over recent years, and an outbreak of new HIV infections in drug users seen in Glasgow in 2015, has once again brought the adequacy of drug-misuse services to the forefront. Although the availability of clean needles and syringes plus opioid substitution programmes have been crucial in the fight to control HIV among drug users in the UK, recently needle exchanges, including one in Glasgow, have been shut down. Or services within them, such as psychological and social interventions assisting changes to injecting behaviours, curtailed. It appears that drug-misuse services have experienced more reduction in funding than any other public health service (National AIDS Trust 2018). The recent rise in deaths of drug users from drug overdoses, and concerns over the drug-related litter left by those injecting in public places, have led to a concerted push for the introduction of drug consumption rooms (DCRs). DCRs are safe, sterile environments in which individuals can inject drugs under supervision, reduce the reuse of unsterile injecting equipment, as well as minimise injury and death from opioid overdoses (Marshall et al. 2011). Although operating successfully across Europe, and in cities such as Vancouver and Sydney (that have high numbers of injecting drug users), in the UK, DCRs are currently illegal, prohibited by the Misuse of Drugs Act, 1971. Once again, a 'harm minimisation' approach is being advocated with calls to change the official UK policy on drug use by amending the Act. However, currently the legal, political and social barriers to DCRs remain substantial (Sherman 2019). Without investment in harm reduction services it is feared that further outbreaks of HIV among drug users are inevitable (National AIDS Trust 2018).

Mass migration, a long-standing part of life in many countries, presents significant health issues in the UK and in continental Europe. A substantial proportion of migrants in European countries have acquired their HIV infection post-migration. They are more likely to receive a delayed HIV diagnosis, suffer stigma and discrimination, and experience significant difficulties accessing HIV prevention and care (Pantazis et al. 2019). Furthermore, female refugees suffer particular isolation and stigma (Bell et al. 2018; Vitale and Ryde 2018), as do refugees ageing with HIV (Terrence Higgins Trust 2017). The UK faces a major challenge to ensure that refugee populations have access to diagnosis and care, and are included in any prevention initiatives, such as those involving access to PrEP.

Finally, stigma – i.e. a personal "attribute that is deeply discrediting" (Goffman 2009) – was a key feature of HIV from the start, being so closely linked to sex, death, and taboo minority groups as it was. PLWH have reported being marked out as inferior, dirty, and unclean (Earnshaw et al. 2013), and stigma has been regarded as a "third wave" of the AIDS epidemic (Earnshaw and Chaudoir 2009; Parker and Aggleton 2003). Early on, PLWH were marked out as 'innocent' or 'guilty' in relation to how they acquired their infection (e.g. anal sex versus blood transfusion), and there was frightening media talk of 'herding up' PLWH (Price and Hsu 1992; Stipp and Kerr 1989; Vanable et al. 2006). With undetectable viral loads preventing HIV from being passed on, and near-normal life expectancy, stigma towards PLWH should surely be a thing of the past. Yet stigma remains a barrier for many PLWH accessing care (Sayles et al. 2009). Stigma can lead to a reluctance to be tested or to engage in HIV treatment, as well as to reduced adherence to medication, opportunistic infections, lower CD4 counts, and reduced quality of life (Green and Platt 1997; Holzemer and Uys 2004; Lee et al. 2002; Link and Phelan 2001; Logie and Gadalla 2009; Sayles et al. 2009; Zierler et al. 2000). Some PLWH have reported a high level of fear of discrimination from healthcare workers who care for them, with breaches of confidentiality not unknown (Green and Platt 1997; Marshall et al. 2017; Steward et al. 2008). There is a considerable way to go achieve zero discrimination by 2030 (a goal of Fast Track Cities), and it is currently unclear how to achieve this laudable ambition.

Examining some of the above issues in more detail below, first we consider some implications of current and future NHS provision, including the tendency towards greater fragmentation and compartmentalisation of services, despite the recent drive towards person-centred care. Next, we look at what it means to not leave any PLWH behind, and touch on the new epidemic of mortality bought on by chemsex, especially relevant to men who have sex with men. Finally, we discuss what success means in terms of prevention.

The changing NHS

The 2019 NHS Long Term Plan focuses on personalised care becoming the bread and butter of patient care, being based on "what matters" to patients and "their individual strengths, needs and preferences" (NHS England 2019, p. 6). Despite the optimistic rhetoric espousing a welcome and renewed focus on person-centredness, there is a sense from our interviewees that there is a way to go to achieve this. As a male charity worker suggested, person-centred care requires strong leadership to establish, maintain, and/or avoid a return to medicalisation:

> *I can see the difference between people with HIV who are much more able to assert what they want, in a nice way, and say they want this, want that, and people being treated for other conditions where the system hasn't quite caught up … In the early days certainly, a very patient-centred model was extraordinary because the only thing you could do was listen and be supportive …I do think that to keep an institution focused on its users, is very, very hard work. The dynamic of an institution tends towards the institution becoming a convenience for the people who work in it primarily. And that you have to work very hard indeed to be resisting that, and it involves very, very clear leadership from the top.*

In terms of mainstreaming, PLWH management is moving from specialised secondary care services to broader primary care management. In taking on this care, there is much HIV-related knowledge that an effective GP needs to know (and is able to do) in the area of HIV, as a male doctor explains in the first quote below. However, PLWH who remember the refusals of some GPs earlier on in the epidemic to care for those with HIV do not always trust mainstreaming. They anticipate discontinuities in care, discrimination, and stigmatising practices, as a Black African man explains:

> *I would say the main problem in Britain is the unwillingness of the medical fraternity to learn about HIV and test …*

> *… most people still aren't out to their GP for one reason or another because they have entrenched views and entrenched feelings, or … we don't want the GP to know because the receptionist is a gossip.*

Nevertheless, there were some encouraging reports that GPs understood the importance of being informed about HIV and treating PLWH with respect and confidentially. By now many GPs have had some exposure to the issues facing PLWH as part of their training, as a hospital doctor stated:

> *Most GPs have now looked after patients when they were housemen or in training and know some HIV patients are on their lists.*

Although there was a sense that primary care might cope, there were lingering doubts, with some PLWH describing their experiences as difficult. Primary care to some people seemed less able to be person-centred, and continuity of care problematic, as articulated by one gay man who has lived with HIV for many decades:

> *And then you've got the cycle of if you're ill, it's like a GP will say, oh that's an HIV-related issue, go and see your clinician. Your clinician will say, no, it's not HIV related, that's your GP, and you can get ping pong … by this point next year I would be really surprised if all of my doctors weren't completely new … knowing that certain people are there, and knowing that you can touch, drop them an email, and they will come back, you can't put a price on that.*

One particular problem with mainstreaming HIV care in the era of austerity is that GP practices themselves are struggling to train and retain enough GPs, with around one in six NHS GP posts remaining vacant (Rosser 2018). Thus, many people have difficulty getting an appointment to see a GP, let alone access a person-centred service. As one HIV doctor put it:

> *… in the last year to 18 months people just can't get in to see their GP, they can't physically. They phone up and say, I have a rash, I have HIV, I'm on drugs and they can't see a GP for two weeks.*

At the same time, an upheaval in primary care is currently underway. For example, there is a move towards other health professionals picking up tasks traditionally done by GPs (e.g. pharmacists, physician associates, social prescribing link workers) and even Artificial Intelligence (AI) becoming involved in diagnosis. For example, the *Babylon GP At Hand* smartphone app which has been promoted by the conservative government, incorporates some AI for diagnosis, and promises NHS GP appointments via mobile phone (Lacobucci 2017). To use the app, patients currently opt out of their GP practice, although they may be able to attend in person to see a GP at certain limited locations. The COVID-19 crisis in early 2020 also resulted in more GP consultations going online to reduce transmissions (Greenhalgh et al. 2020). It remains unclear how such rapid changes will impact on PLWH. For example, social prescribing 'link workers' could potentially spend more time with PLWH, and help those who are isolated with complex physical and mental health issues (Drinkwater et al. 2019). However, other problems, including timely and joined-up care, do not have easy solutions.

In parallel with the general impact of austerity on public services, the specific effect of the implementation in England of the Lansley reforms (see Chapter 5), separating the funding of treatment which is centrally led, from public health services funded locally, is likely to have adverse consequences. The 'Public Health England' organisation was created in 2013, and public health functions were transferred to local authorities. These public services include not just prevention in the strictest sense, but also the funding of substance misuse and sexual health services. Between 2016 and 2018, funding for substance misuse was cut by £81 million (11%) and sexual health services by £55 million (9%) (Appleby 2018). Subsequently, the chief executives of the National AIDS Trust, the Terrence Higgins Trust, the chair of the British HIV Association, and the president of the British Association for Sexual Health and HIV stated publicly that, "We are on the verge of a crisis in sexual health services ... A plan to reverse the damage done and to protect public and prevent avoidable consequences is desperately needed" (Gold et al. 2018).

Not leaving anyone behind

As highlighted in this book, there is always a danger that the extraordinary treatment successes might overshadow social problems that are harder to define. The complex health needs of the increasing numbers of ageing PLWH as mentioned above, along with their co-morbidities, require us to focus on improving long-term well-being, not just viral suppression (Safreed-Harmon et al. 2019). There are other groups of socially vulnerable PLWH in the UK, particularly the victims of austerity policies. Despite being the world's fifth largest economy, ideologically driven UK government policies since 2010 have taken their toll: 20 % of the UK population live in poverty, and there is a proliferation of food banks and homelessness, as well as a near collapse of the entire legal aid system (Alston 2019). Unsurprisingly, Michael Marmot's report published in 2020, 10 years after the landmark *Fair Society, Healthy Lives Review*, found that the gap in health between the poorest and wealthiest had widened in the UK, with life expectancy stalled since 2010 for the first time in 100 years, and some groups (e.g. the poorest women) experiencing an actual decline in life expectancy (Marmot et al. 2020).

The re-medicalisation of HIV occurred at the same time as austerity policies, leading to a decimation of UK HIV organisations (Dalton 2018). However, disadvantaged and vulnerable PLWH continue to need assistance to manage their HIV health conditions and lives (Gardiner 2018). While discourses about healthy ageing are generally available to all PLWH, we know from the research cited above that well-being and health are unequally distributed in the population. For example, many older PLWH in rural areas to this day are still subject to the high levels of gossip, social isolation, homonegativity, shame, and lack of social support characteristic of the early epidemic (Quinn et al. 2019). Additionally, the cohort of PLWH who went through the early traumas outlined in this book may have entirely different issues to contend with compared to people being diagnosed now, as a gay man with HIV noted:

> ... they actually are the ones that have suffered the most because there's a lot of issues that they carry forward ... The issues of survivor guilt, the issues, they lost their, all their friends, partners etc., and the services are more and more being geared towards today where you've got somebody that quite literally, oh I'm HIV positive. OK, go from one room to the other, get a set of pills, go home and take them. It's a very much more

relaxed, casual, straightforward [thing].

Not surprisingly, the move to less frequent appointments for HIV, while fine for some, like many of the newly diagnosed, may be experienced as an abandonment by others, at least in the short term, as one community nurse noted:

> *Well I think again people feel quite left because there were, they did have quite frequent hospital appointments, and now it's once every six months or once every six months or once a year...*

For PLWH diagnosed early on in the epidemic, there is a sense that as their original practitioners retire, they are losing long-standing relationships which in the past were so reassuring and important for their well-being. A gay man living with HIV put it this way:

> *But it was having him [psychiatrist] there in the background in case anything went wrong helped tremendously, not so much with me but with [partner] because he's been a bit more mentally precarious than I have. So, and of course now he's gone, we feel he's gone. He retired, that's fine. Since he's gone we've had – he went in December last year – we're on our third locum psychiatrist.*

As people with HIV get older, social care in later life becomes more pressing. However, many studies have concluded that for many older LGBTQ people, particularly those with HIV, at a minimum there are perceptions of (if not actual) homophobia, and erasure of sexuality and social differences in social care environments (Kneale et al. 2019). Some men who have sex with men in our sample were concerned about the lack of social policy and planning, with a perceived gap in service provision where stigma was thought to be likely. What happens, for example, if same-sex relationships are formed/displayed in residential care? How accepting will staff be? There are fears about the details of care, including whether adherence to HIV medication regimes is achievable, as a doctor working in HIV noted:

> *But as our [cohort] of what, of nearly 100,000 [PLWH] gets older, gets forgetful, gets demented what's going to happen, and how are people living with HIV going to fare in nursing homes? Are they going to still be given their medicine on time, every day?*

In an era of austerity, many of those diagnosed in the 80s and 90s in the UK have now faced up to losing their disability benefits despite not being fit for work. Here, it can be difficult for agencies to understand that issues like fatigue, multiple morbidities and mental health problems do not necessarily show up in viral loads and CD4 counts, as one psychiatrist working with PLWH highlighted:

> *So one of the patients said ... my CD4 may be good but what about the whole list of symptoms that I have that I live with ... a lot of grief and lot of the diarrhoeas and you know fatigue ... they have a constant battle with social services in terms of the money*

and the benefits and I think that's a big thing they just feel that they have to prove it to other people that … They're unwell and the numbers like the viral load and the CD4 count is not a reflection of their quality of life and what they can or can't do …

In this climate of fear and misperception, we heard anecdotal reports of people stopping their medication in a desperate attempt to avoid having their funds dry up, as a community-based nurse claimed,

People were stopping taking their drugs so that they could get their benefits.

Another finding of our research was the concern about chemsex among gay men, including how it accounted for deaths in the post-HIV-crisis era. Importantly, not all men who engage in sexualised drug use are dissatisfied with their behaviours, and sex with substances is considered by many men to be 'ubiquitous' in gay culture (Ahmed et al. 2016). Thus, one of the challenges for professionals is distinguishing between culturally sanctioned use and denial when things go wrong. Many men who have sex with men, who engage in sexualised drug use, do not necessarily see themselves as misusing drugs. Thus, they can find it hard to relate to mainstream drug services, as the psychiatrist notes in the first quote below. Nevertheless, those who work in the HIV field can doubt their own suitability in assisting men with drug-related problems, as the doctor remarks in the second quote:

… this is a group who would not see themselves as belonging to the substance misuse side … especially the chemsex side … there aren't very good services, there's no good places we can send them to. So, I think I've taken on more of that work here as much as I can …

So, if somebody has become terribly paranoid and upset and distressed and agitated after their crystal meth experience, I'm not the best person to look after them, they need people who are experienced in mental health and in drug rehab…

Continuing prevention work

One of the concerns following the success of the Fast Track Cities[1] approach, with London being the first city to meet a 95–95–95 target, is that funding for HIV will be cut further. Nevertheless, London has signed up for no new infections, no preventable deaths, zero stigma and the highest quality of life for PLWH by 2030 (Anon 2020). This is a complex task requiring high levels of coordination to diagnose HIV infections as early as possible, treat HIV infections rapidly, along with supporting excellent and innovative approaches to preventative work. Our participants were keen to point out the ongoing challenges, as first an HIV doctor and then a gay activist living with HIV remarked:

There are 10,000 people living in the UK with undiagnosed HIV, we've got to find them, treat them.

Education is a challenge that needs to be repeated and repeated, and it is ongoing as every generation becomes … sexually active.

The relevant voluntary HIV sector organisations with all their accumulated expertise are under immense financial pressures, and many are closing. Ironically, more success (as measured by reduced HIV infections and illness) is likely to be accompanied by a further dwindling interest in HIV. One HIV doctor drew a contrast between clinics then and now to show that patients themselves are less invested in HIV:

> *If you come to a Monday afternoon clinic now, 30 years ago there'd have been people there with visible KS, people with high volume diarrhoea with drips and sitting in wheelchairs and visibly a really sick population. Now people are coming in and going, look can the pharmacy get on with it, I've got to get back to work …*

The effectiveness of PrEP, including the renewed activism around it, is another success story as mentioned above. Certainly, in London, the dramatic reductions in infections in recent years coincided with community campaigning to increase PrEP uptake, and there is a sense that PrEP has reenergised the HIV sector following the decline in community activism over the years. A male activist said:

> *… because [PrEP is] where the new energy is coming from, because us oldies, dinosaurs, we won't be around for very long, for much longer. I'm getting tired, I'm seeing signs of ageing myself, I haven't got the energy I used to have.*

Nevertheless, there was also a sense that community activism can also spring up in unexpected places, such as in terms of the needs of those people growing older with HIV, as an activist in his 50s said:

> *So I got into a bit, a little bit of HIV and ageing activism with [a charity] … So I've become a little bit more, dabbled in a bit of activism, a bit of politics I suppose over the last couple of years, and that's where I am.*

And despite the success of PrEP, there were concerns that this approach could eventually reveal its limitations, as one man living with HIV noted:

> *I worry about resistance possibly with these people and stuff, and maybe, I don't know, maybe that it's developing, going to develop potentially a new set of HIV problems, I don't know.*

There was also a sense among some that another infectious epidemic may appear on the horizon at some stage. While COVID-19 is not specifically transmitted by sex, it is highly infectious and transmitted by close contact, which includes sex. So just as HIV appeared to come from nowhere, once again we need to find a way to prevent – as well as cope with – novel infections. One HIV doctor asked:

> *… how are MSM and heterosexuals both and other people of the whole LGBT community going to express themselves sexually and experiment, be highly sexual, but at the same time encourage people to stay safe so that we don't get whatever's coming next?*

Conclusion

The HIV pandemic has shown how what was initially perceived as a major global threat, with impacts across the world, came under greater control, not as the result of a miracle cure, but as a consequence of the hard work and collaboration of people with HIV, volunteers, healthcare workers, researchers and key policy makers. International collaboration was an essential element in the process of learning about HIV and how to deal with it. We hope we have done justice in this book by giving a voice to the many people who fought hard to ensure that the human rights and social needs of PLWH and their families were met. The voices of key people involved in the HIV epidemic in the UK are presented in our book. Sadly, we lost many people to HIV along the way, and HIV has not yet been eradicated, although the technical means to do so are available. Access to care and prevention remains a problem in many parts of the world including the UK, as does stigma and discrimination. The will and determination to tackle these structural obstacles need to be renewed by each generation. We hope that our participant stories help to ensure that the achievements of the previous decades are not forgotten. We hope that we have inspired new generations to find new ways to cope with the challenges still posed by HIV and by epidemics yet to come.

Note

1 Fast-Track Cities is a global collaboration of cities particularly affected by HIV, with partners like the United Nations Programme on HIV/AIDS (UNAIDS) and International Association of Providers of AIDS Care (IAPAC) to end HIV by 2030. The aim is zero stigma by 2030, and that 95% of PLWH become aware of their status; 95% get sustained antiretroviral therapy (ART); and 95% achieving viral suppression.

References

Ahmed, A-K, Weatherburn, P, Reid, D, Hickson, F, Torres-Rueda, S, Steinberg, P, and Bourne, A (2016) Social norms related to combining drugs and sex ("chemsex") among gay men in South London. *International Journal of Drug Policy*, 38, 29–35. https://doi.org/10.1016/j.drugpo.2016.10.007

Alston, P (2019) Visit to the United Kingdom of Great Britain and Northern Ireland: Report of the special rapporteur on extreme poverty and human rights. *Human Rights Council, United Nations*. https://digitallibrary.un.org/record/3806308?ln=en

Anon (2020) Time to PrEP for zero HIV transmissions in the UK? *The Lancet HIV*, 7(3), E149. https://doi.org/10.1016/S2352-3018(20)30037-0.

Appleby, J (2018) This is what's happening to NHS spending on public health. *BMJ*, 363, k4869. doi:https://doi.org/10.1136/bmj.k4869

Bell, E, Hale, F, Kwardem, L, Laycock, D, Lennon, J, and Stevenson, J (2018) *Women and HIV: invisible no longer.* London, Sophia Forum & Terrence Higgins Trust.

Criado-Perez, C (2019) *Invisible women: Exposing data bias in a world designed for men.* London, Chatto & Windus.

Dalton, D (2018) Cutting the ribbon? Austerity measures and the problems faced by the HIV third sector. In P Rushton and C Donavan (Eds), *Austerity policies* (pp. 173–195). Cham, Palgrave Macmillan.

de Iongh, A, Redding, D, and Leonard, H (2019) New personalised care plan for the NHS. *BMJ*, 364, l470. doi:10.1136/bmj.l470

Drinkwater, C, Wildman, J, and Moffatt, S (2019) Social prescribing. *BMJ*, 364, l1285. doi:10.1136/bmj.l1285

Earnshaw, VA, and Chaudoir, SR (2009) From conceptualizing to measuring HIV stigma: a review of HIV stigma mechanism measures. *AIDS and Behavior*, 13(6), 1160.

Earnshaw, VA, Smith, LR, Chaudoir, SR, Amico, KR, and Copenhaver, MM (2013) HIV stigma mechanisms and well-being among PLWH: a test of the HIV stigma framework. *AIDS and Behavior*, 17(5), 1785–1795.

Gardiner, B (2018) Grit and stigma: Gay men ageing with HIV in regional Queensland. *Journal of Sociology*, 54(2), 214–225. doi:10.1177/1440783318766162

Goffman, E (2009) *Stigma: notes on the management of spoiled identity*. Cliffs, N.J: Prentice-Hall.

Gold, D, Green, I, Orkin, C, and Carlin, E (2018, 14th January 2020) The big issue: sexual health services must be protected to prevent a crisis. *Guardian*. https://www.theguardian.com/news/2018/jan/14/big-issue-sexual-health-services-must-be-protected

Green, G, and Platt, S (1997) Fear and loathing in health care settings reported by people with HIV. *Sociology of Health & Illness*, 19(1), 70–92.

Greenhalgh, T, Wherton, J, Shaw, S, and Morrison, C (2020) Video consultations for covid-19. *BMJ*, 368, m998. doi:10.1136/bmj.m998

Holzemer, WL, and Uys, LR (2004) Managing AIDS stigma. *SAHARA-J: Journal of Social Aspects of HIV/AIDS*, 1(3), 165–174.

Kneale, D, Henley, J, Thomas, J, and French, R (2019) Inequalities in older LGBT people's health and care needs in the United Kingdom: a systematic scoping review. *Ageing and Society*, 1–23. doi:10.1017/S0144686X19001326

Lacobucci, G (2017) London GP clinic sees big jump in patient registrations after Babylon app launch. *BMJ*, 359, j5908. doi:10.1136/bmj.j5908

Lee, RS, Kochman, A, and Sikkema, KJ (2002) Internalized stigma among people living with HIV-AIDS. *AIDS and Behavior*, 6(4), 309–319.

Link, BG, and Phelan, JC (2001) Conceptualizing stigma. *Annual Review of Sociology*, 27(1), 363–385.

Logie, C, and Gadalla, T (2009) Meta-analysis of health and demographic correlates of stigma towards people living with HIV. *AIDS Care*, 21(6), 742–753.

Marmot, M, Allen, J, Boyce, T, Goldblatt, P, and Morrison, J (2020) *Health equity in England: The Marmot Review 10 years on*. London, British Medical Journal. 368: m693.

Marshall, BD, Milloy, MJ, Wood, E, Montaner, JS, and Kerr, T (2011) Reduction in overdose mortality after the opening of North America's first medically supervised safer injecting facility: a retrospective population-based study. *The Lancet*, 377(9775), 1429–1437.

Marshall, AS, Brewington, KM, Kathryn Allison, M, Haynes, TF, and Zaller, ND (2017) Measuring HIV-related stigma among healthcare providers: a systematic review. *AIDS Care*, 29(11), 1337–1345.

Nagington, M, and Sandset, T (2020) Putting the NHS England on trial: uncertainty-as-power, evidence and the controversy of PrEP in England. *Medical Humanities*, 46, 176–179. doi:10.1136/medhum-2019-011780

National AIDS Trust (2018) *Policy Briefing: HIV Outbreak in Glasgow – more needs to be done*. https://www.nat.org.uk/sites/default/files/HIV_outbreak_in_glasgow_1.pdf

NHS England (2019) *The NHS long term plan*. London: NHS England.

Pantazis, N, Thomadakis, C, del Amo, J, Alvarez-del Arco, D, Burns, FM, Fakoya, I, and Touloumi, G (2019) Determining the likely place of HIV acquisition for migrants in Europe combining subject-specific information and biomarkers data. *Statistical Methods in Medical Research*, 28(7), 1979–1997. doi:10.1177/0962280217746437

Parker, R, and Aggleton, P (2003) HIV and AIDS-related stigma and discrimination: a conceptual framework and implications for action. *Social Science & Medicine*, 57(1), 13–24.

Price, V, and Hsu, M-L (1992) Public opinion about AIDS policies. The role of misinformation and attitudes toward homosexuals. *Public Opinion Quarterly*, 56(1), 29–52.

Quinn, KG, Murphy, MK, Nigogosyan, Z, and Petroll, AE (2019) Stigma, isolation and depression among older adults living with HIV in rural areas. *Ageing and Society*, 40, 1–19. doi:10.1017/S0144686X18001782

Rose, N (2007) *The politics of life itself: Biomedicine, power, and subjectivity in the twenty-first century*. Oxford, Princeton University Press.

Rosenfeld, D, Ridge, D, and Catalan, J (2019) Ageing with HIV. In S Westwood (Ed.), *Ageing, diversity and equality: social justice perspectives* (pp. 259–275). London, Routledge.

Rosser, E (2018) Revealed: GP vacancy rates rocket with one in six roles unfilled. *Pulse*. Retrieved from http://www.pulsetoday.co.uk/partners-/practice-business/revealed-gp-vacancy-rates-rocket-with-one-in-six-roles-unfilled/20036995.article

Safreed-Harmon, K, Anderson, J, Azzopardi-Muscat, N, Behrens, GMN, d'Arminio Monforte, A, Davidovich, U, … Lazarus, JV (2019) Reorienting health systems to care for people with HIV beyond viral suppression. *The Lancet HIV*, 6(12), e869-e877. doi: https://doi.org/10.1016/S2352-3018(19)30334-0

Sayles, JN, Wong, MD, Kinsler, JJ, Martins, D, and Cunningham, WE (2009) The association of stigma with self-reported access to medical care and antiretroviral therapy adherence in persons living with HIV/AIDS. *Journal of General Internal Medicine*, 24(10), 1101.

Sherman, S (2019) Overdose prevention sites and heroin assisted treatment. *British Medical Journal*, 366: l5437.

Sherr, L, Molloy, A, Macedo, A, Croome, N, and Johnson, M (2016) Ageing and menopause considerations for women with HIV in the UK. *Journal of Virus Eradication*, 2(4), 215.

Steward, WT, Herek, GM, Ramakrishna, J, Bharat, S, Chandy, S, Wrubel, J, and Ekstrand, ML (2008) HIV-related stigma: adapting a theoretical framework for use in India. *Social Science & Medicine*, 67(8), 1225–1235.

Stipp, H, and Kerr, D (1989) Determinants of public opinion about AIDS. *Public Opinion Quarterly*, 53(1), 98–106.

Terrence Higgins Trust (2017) *Uncharted territory: a report into the first generation growing older with HIV*. London, THT.

Vanable, PA, Carey, MP, Blair, DC, and Littlewood, RA (2006) Impact of HIV-related stigma on health behaviors and psychological adjustment among HIV-positive men and women. *AIDS and Behavior*, 10(5), 473–482.

Vitale, A, and Ryde, J (2018) Exploring risk factors affecting the mental health of refugee women living with HIV. *International Journal of Environmental Research and Public Health*, 15(10), 2326.

Zierler, S, Cunningham, WE, Andersen, R, Shapiro, MF, Nakazono, T, Morton, S, … St Clair, P (2000) Violence victimization after HIV infection in a US probability sample of adult patients in primary care. *American Journal of Public Health*, 90(2), 208.

Postscript: What can the HIV epidemic tell us about COVID-19?

As we are finalising the manuscript for this book, we are about 12 weeks into the 2020 UK lockdown for COVID-19. We cannot help but make links between HIV and the novel coronavirus (SARS-CoV-2).

HIV and the coronavirus seemed to appear suddenly on the scene, although both were spreading in the community before they were recognised. Some argued that HIV could have been predicted, as Larry Kramer had in the US, and the likelihood of another flu-like pandemic had been anticipated by many. Denial of its impact or minimisation of the risks it posed, was the first response in the UK and US, both in relation to HIV, and now with COVID-19, followed by a public response of fear and stigma. For HIV it was gay men early on who were blamed for the virus, with some people living with HIV (PLWH) being driven from their homes and hounded in the tabloid newspapers, with calls to 'herd them up'. Now it is the Chinese who are blamed for the failed approaches to the pandemic in some Western democracies like the US, with its president referring to the virus as the 'Chinese virus', while making unsubstantiated claims that the virus came from a laboratory in China. There was discrimination against older and disabled people, those in care homes, as well as their carers (who were left without personal protective equipment), suggesting that such people were somehow dispensable members of society.

We know from HIV that stigma only drives epidemics underground, making it all that much harder to do the vital work of testing for the virus, tracing contacts, isolating the virus so it cannot infect others, and encouraging people to acknowledge their infection and come forward for treatment. Indeed, *Fast Track Cities*,[1] realising that stigma stands in the way of ending the HIV epidemic, has set a target of zero discrimination for HIV by 2030, as part of its strategy to end HIV once and for all. A virus is a biological entity, it does not discriminate, it does not have a morality. It will instead mercilessly exploit stigma and any other flaws in our public health approaches. As we write this, we celebrate with New Zealand, who have announced the virtual elimination of the coronavirus. Their approach was always based on coming together as a community, moving quickly based on the public health science, and isolating the virus – by hunting it down ruthlessly – while caring for the people of New Zealand. South Korea also had an excellent public health response. That was until stigma against men who have sex with men (MSM) led to those men giving false identities, undermining an otherwise efficient track and trace system, giving rise to spikes of new COVID-19.

Apart from the importance of dealing with stigma, HIV and its history provide many other relevant lessons for facing the challenges raised by COVID-19. We would like to focus in this postscript on prevention of its spread, treatment, and dealing with death in our death denying culture.

Prevention of coronavirus spread requires a combination of political and public health decisions, and the engagement of individuals from the populations at risk in responding positively to such recommendations. Testing, contact tracing, and isolation are clear examples of the political and public health actions needed. At an individual level, behaviour changes, such as physical and social distancing, 'contact clustering',[2] or 'social bubbles' will only work if they are adequately explained and seriously adopted and evaluated. This was the way safer-sex behaviour and condom use were advocated to reduce the risk of transmission of HIV, against other approaches, such as 'negotiated safety'[3] and 'zero grazing',[4] which were never properly evaluated. Changes at an individual level, however, require taking into account health inequalities and vulnerabilities which have a major impact on the ability of individuals to change their behaviour.

Preventing transmission by means of a vaccine is often mentioned as the ultimate solution to the COVID-19 pandemic. There are positive noises currently from various quarters, but there is a cautionary note from the HIV epidemic – the UK and other countries poured huge amounts of money and expertise into HIV vaccine research in the mid-80s to no avail, and this year we witnessed yet another HIV vaccine failure.

The history of HIV research also resonates with the Black Lives Matter protests that are currently sweeping the globe. We are reminded of the case of an HIV treatment trial that compared the efficacy of the prospective drug with a placebo in preventing infection to infants born to women with HIV. This trial was conducted in Africa, where many infected babies were born to those receiving the placebo. In the West, HIV activists had secured a voice ensuring no one would be disadvantaged in clinical trials, and a similar trial was carried out with no placebo arm. This kind of discriminatory devaluing of (Black) lives must never be repeated for COVID-19.

When it comes to looking for COVID-19 treatments, science works slowly and incrementally. Like now, in the early days of the HIV epidemic there was much talk of finding the right treatment, with individual drugs rumoured to be on the horizon. But effective treatments are likely to take time to discover, develop, trial, distribute, and make widely available on a global scale. The first antiretroviral for HIV (AZT), much heralded in the 1980s did seem to bring some respite, together with difficult side effects. But, only a few years later in 1993 it became clear from research trials that AZT brought no long-term improvements on mortality, nor did it slow the onset of AIDS. Since then, medication has become more effective, but only after the recognition that a combination of drugs was required to interfere with HIV replication so that it could not mutate and develop resistance to the effective medications. With the application of effective treatments, our book uncovered a

'Lazarus Slowly Effect': those PLWH with depleted immune systems came back to life, slowly, but it was heartbreakingly too late for other people who literally saw the good news, but it did not work for them.

Although in the UK HIV treatments became available, fear of discrimination kept some from coming forward to receive them. There is the very real risk that treatment success in COVID-19 will again side-line more marginalised people. COVID-19 is not the great equaliser – it affects the vulnerable and disadvantaged most, including Black and minority ethnic people. With HIV treatment success, marginalised people remained so, with ongoing health problems, little suitable work available, few savings, and poor mental health. With COVID-19, those with the least resources – including poorly paid key workers – are not able to work from home or self-isolate like many in the middle-classes can do to protect themselves. Additionally, it is not currently clear to what extent any successful treatments or vaccines will be made equitably available on a global scale.

As our understanding of the impact of COVID-19 increases, it is becoming clear that there are complex longer-term consequences, both physical and psychological, which will need addressing. Treatment for COVID-19 must include not just medication, but also the involvement of multidisciplinary teams, and the use of a person-centred approach, as the care of people with HIV demonstrated. The psychological impact on healthcare workers of dealing with many patients with COVID-19 is now starting to become apparent. There are also the relatives of those who did not survive to consider, who had little or no contact with loved ones as they succumbed to the virus. In the case of HIV, activists – both those infected and those affected by it – played a fundamental role in highlighting the needs and problems faced by people with the infection and fighting stigma, as well as developing effective community support responses and organisations. There are hints of this earlier HIV activism in relation to COVID-19, which we hope will only grow in future.

We live in a death-denying society. In the weeks prior to writing this postscript, it was as if we were losing a passenger airliner of people daily in the UK, but we were unable to process the loss. Behind the daily tally of deaths, real lives were being lost, but the invisibility of suffering was remarkable. Yet each lost life had a story to tell, including the stories from those that loved them. COVID-19 deaths remained out of sight, they are a mystery to us. We learnt from HIV that it was important publicly to commemorate and celebrate the lives of the dead, such as via the AIDS Quilt, with each panel celebrating a person's life in moving ways. This helped to humanise stigmatised people, and drew attention to the need to fight HIV. With the spectre of death hanging over us again, lockdown has been a retreat for some, allowing people to re-evaluate their lives, recognising what is important, and what they could let go of. HIV and the certainty of death also propelled communities – including health professionals – to live more fulfilled lives. However, as we show in this book, any understanding of the importance of acknowledging death and bereavement can soon be forgotten. The status quo is denial, and this is not helped by COVID-19 restrictions placed on funerals through fears of further virus transmission. It is important to help people continue to talk about death and conditions such as COVID-19, if people are to better process the trauma, the loss, and live well.

HIV showed us the importance of telling and sharing in human stories and discussing the issues involved, as a vital first step to attracting people's interest and understanding of the underlying issues, and gaining political traction for support. The heads of the UK and the US governments were both slow to act on the emergence of HIV. Back then many UK politicians seemed to think HIV would remain localised to the US, just as they thought COVID-19 would remain in China, or at least in Asia. Governments were fatally slow to respond to both HIV and COVID-19 but with both, remarkable people stepped forward and tried to inform and caution – gay men with HIV, Chinese doctors in Wuhan, and various public health experts in the UK for COVID-19. In the 1980s it took the pressure of gay activists, frontline clinicians and public health experts for the politicians to act, to collaborate and deal humanely (rather than reactively) with the extraordinary existential threat posed by HIV. We can see the same struggle with COVID-19 now, and this pressure from key individuals (e.g. public health experts, patients telling their stories in the media, care workers and clinicians on the frontline) was critical in forcing better responses to COVID-19 in the UK and elsewhere. Both HIV and COVID-19 teach us that as much as being about a biological entity, pandemics are shaped by social circumstances, and the choices we make in addressing it are critical. Politicians have to be educated, lobbied, and otherwise encouraged to respond appropriately.

Initially, with no effective treatments for HIV, the NHS and social care workers could only focus on the whole-person needs of those ill and dying. HIV care thus became an incubator for a radical re-imagining of health and social care that elevated patient experience in a way that was without precedent for a state health service. A change that would anticipate – and gradually help usher in an NHS discourse about personalisation – including the idea that patients could be more involved in – and be allowed increasing control of – their care. Once the threat of a global spread of HIV was appreciated, NHS care for those with HIV was well funded. Now, with recent cuts to health and social care budgets, and service reorganisation, there is a drift back from the gains associated with the personal-care approach achieved in HIV. With COVID-19, funds only gradually seem to be becoming available to carers with provision of personal protective equipment, and properly funded testing and tracing. As with the HIV epidemic, the temptation will be for a drift back from the gains, towards the status quo, once this crisis is over. Clapping and saying how wonderful NHS and social care workers are, is the easy bit. This needs to be the start of a more comprehensive review of service provision, and improvements in the status of frontline health and social care workers. The failure to invest in a UK safe blood supply, although agreed to be necessary, led to transmissions of HIV through transfusions and factor VIII. Similarly, although a mock-up of a pandemic in 2017 indicated the unpreparedness of UK to respond well, there was no apparent implementation of findings. The result has been the unnecessary loss of tens of thousands of lives. Each of them had more living to do.

London, 26 June 2020

Notes

1 Fast-Track Cities is a global collaboration of cities particularly affected by HIV, with partners like the United Nations Programme on HIV/AIDS (UNAIDS) and International Association of Providers of AIDS Care (IAPAC) to end HIV by 2030.

2 'Contact clustering' is the formation of quarantine 'bubbles', a concept introduced by Prof Stefan Flasche, LSHTM, to refer to a group of people with close contact within the cluster, but social distancing outside.

3 'Negotiated safety' was an approach to reduce transmission in MSM couples by advising condom unprotected sex within the couple, provided each partner agreed to be safe with other sexual partners.

4 'Zero grazing' was advocated in some African communities to reduce heterosexual transmission of HIV: men were advised to have regular partners and not 'graze' freely outside of those partners.

Appendix

The participants' demographics, roles, and where appropriate HIV status, are given below:

Table A Participant data

		N (%)	N (%)	N (%)
		Male	*Female*	*Total*
		36 (68)	*17 (32)*	*53*
Ethnicity	Caucasian	35 (97)	13 (76)	48 (91)
	African/Afro-Caribbean	1 (3)	2 (12)	3 (6)
	South East Asian/Indian	0 (0)	2 (12)	2 (4)
HIV status	Positive	19 (53)	2 (12)	21 (40)
	Negative or untested	17 (47)	15 (88)	32 (60)
Role★	Health professional	14 (39)	10 (59)	24 (45)
	Activist	9 (25)	0 (0)	9 (17)
	Charity worker	3 (8)	1 (6)	4 (8)
	PLWH	19 (53)	2 (12)	21 (40)
	Other★★	6 (17)	4 (24)	10 (19)
Mode of transmission★★★	MSM	14 (39)	0 (0)	14 (26)
	Heterosexual	1 (3)	2 (12)	3 (6)
	Injecting drug use	2 (6)	0 (0)	2 (4)
	Haemophilia	2 (6)	0 (0)	2 (4)

★ Participants may have more than one role
★★ Journalist/Politician/Clergy/Academic/Policy Maker
★★★ Self-reported as most likely

Index

For Product Safety Concerns and Information please contact our EU
representative GPSR@taylorandfrancis.com
Taylor & Francis Verlag GmbH, Kaufingerstraße 24, 80331 München, Germany

www.ingramcontent.com/pod-product-compliance
Ingram Content Group UK Ltd.
Pitfield, Milton Keynes, MK11 3LW, UK
UKHW021453080625
459435UK00012B/484